THE APPENDICITIS DIET PLAN FOR BEGINNERS

Savor Over 100 Superfoods for Recovery, Prevention of Complications, and Quick Healing After an Appendectomy

Gale Nicole RDN

COPYRIGHT PAGE

© 2024 by Gale Nicole RDN. All rights reserved. No part of this publication may be reproduced, distributed, or transmitted in any form or by any means, including photocopying, recording, or other electronic or mechanical methods, without the prior written permission of the author, except in the case of brief quotations embodied in critical reviews and certain other noncommercial uses permitted by copyright law.

The information provided in this cookbook is for general informational purposes only. It is not intended as a substitute for professional medical advice, diagnosis, or treatment. Always seek the advice of your dietician/doctor/physician or other qualified health care provider with any questions you may have regarding a medical condition.

The author and publisher are not responsible for any effects or consequences resulting from the use of the recipes or information presented in this diet cookbook.

Contents

COPYRIGHT PAGE 2

Contents 4

ALL YOU NEED TO KNOW ABOUT APPENDIX 1

    What Is Appendicitis? 9

    Causes and Risk Factors That May Predispose You to Appendicitis 12

    Do I Have Appendicitis? Symptoms to Check for and Diagnostic Evaluations 17

    Treatment and Prevention Strategies for Managing Appendicitis 30

APPENDICITIS PRE-SURGERY DIET 39

    Foods to Avoid to Prevent Worsening Symptoms 42

    Pre-Surgery Hydration Tips 49

Role of Low-Fiber Foods in Reducing Inflammation 53

POST-SURGERY DIET: HEALING AND RECOVERY 62

Staying Hydrated for Digestive Wellness 70

Managing Digestive Sensitivities Post-Surgery 76

Constipation After Surgery: Tips for Relief 81

APPENDICITIS DIET RECIPES YOU MUST TRY 86

BREAKFAST RECIPES TO START YOUR DAY RIGHT 87

Creamy cherry smoothie (low Fiber) 87

Aloo masala (Low Fiber) 88

Eggy devils (Low Fiber) 91

Basil zoodle frittata (Low Fiber) 93

Eastern baked eggs (Low Fiber) 95

Creamy coconut apple porridge (Low Fiber) . 98

Curried carrot soup (Low Fiber) 100

Potato soup with apples and Brie (Low fiber) 103

Peanut Butter & Chia Berry Jam English Muffin 106

Raspberry-Peach-Mango Smoothie Bowl 107

Spinach-Avocado Smoothie 110

Peanut Butter-Banana English Muffin 111

Blueberry Almond Chia Pudding 112

Raspberry Yogurt Cereal Bowl 114

DELICIOUS LUNCH RECIPES SUGGESTION FOR YOU 116

Low Fiber Lunch Recipe Suggestions 116

Baked cod with lemon and capers 116

Balsamic feta chicken 118

White sea bass with dill relish 120

Thai peanut beef 122

Swordfish with roasted lemons 124

Sweet potato souffle 126

Barbecued pork tenderloin 128

High Fiber Lunch Recipe Suggestions 132

Avocado Toast with Burrata 132

Chicken, Avocado & Quinoa Bowls with Herb Dressing 133

Meal-Prep Roasted Vegetable Bowls with Pesto 138

Halloumi Grain Bowls With Figs and Charred Lemon Dressing 140

Superfood Lentil Salad 143

Turkey-Pumpkin Chili 147

Sweet Potato and Kale Tortilla Soup 149

Creamy Miso White Bean Soup 153

DINNER RECIPES SUGGESTION FOR YOU .. 156

Low Fiber Recipe Suggestions 156

    Blackened sole 156

    Broiled grouper with teriyaki sauce 158

    Chicken Parmesan 160

    Fish Veracruz 162

    Grilled salmon 164

    Pork tenderloin with apples and blue cheese 166

    Roasted salmon with maple glaze 168

High Fiber Recipe Suggestions 170

    Easy Pea & Spinach Carbonara 170

    Quinoa Chickpea Salad with Roasted Red Pepper Hummus Dressing 173

    Sautéed Broccoli with Peanut Sauce 174

Loaded Gentle Black Bean Nacho Soup.........177

Cheesy Spinach-&-Artichoke Stuffed Spaghetti Squash..................178

Spaghetti & Chicken Meatballs with No-Cook Tomato Sauce..................181

SNACK AND DESSERT RECIPE SUGGESTIONS
..................184

Raspberry-Jam Bites..................184

Blueberry-Lemon Energy Balls..................186

Banana Bran Muffins..................188

Kale Chips..................191

Chocolate-Peppermint Energy Balls..................192

Pineapple Spinach Smoothie..................194

Peanut Butter and Banana Breakfast Sandwich
..................195

Blueberry-Pecan Energy Balls..................197

Bagel Gone Bananas 199

Cranberry-Almond Energy Balls 200

Pumpkin-Oatmeal Muffins 201

Apple Pie Energy Balls 203

Rosemary-Garlic Pecans 205

APPENDICITIS DIET FOR CHILDREN 207

Transitioning to the Appendicitis Diet 212

Preparing for your appointment 215

1
ALL YOU NEED TO KNOW ABOUT APPENDIX

The appendix is a finger-like tube in the lower right part of the abdomen. It is attached to the cecum, which is the first part of the large intestine, near the end of the small intestine.

Its role has long been a mystery, but some experts believe they're closer to understanding its function. The appendix is perhaps best known because of appendicitis. This is a fairly common medical condition that can happen if the appendix becomes blocked or inflamed.

Where Is Your Appendix?

Your appendix is located in the lower right part of your abdomen, in an area that doctors refer to as McBurney's point. If applying pressure on McBurney's point results in pain or tenderness, your doctor may suspect you have appendicitis.

The finger-shaped appendix is attached to a part of your large intestine called the cecum — a small pouch typically considered to be the beginning of the large intestine.

What Is the Function of the Appendix?

The muscles lining your GI tract, along with the hormones and enzymes that the system produces, allow your GI tract to break down and process food. Your appendix doesn't directly help with digestion either. Furthermore, removal of the organ doesn't appear to have any negative health consequences.

So what exactly is its role? There are a few theories.

A Vestigial Organ

For many years, scientists believed the appendix was a vestigial organ — one that lost its original function through centuries of evolution.

Researchers thought that no other mammals had an appendix, aside from our closest ape relatives.

What's more, the cecum (a part of the large intestine) of plant-eating mammals is far larger than it is in humans.

On this basis, Charles Darwin theorized that our distant ancestors also had large ceca, which allowed them to dine on leaves like the herbivores of today.

But as these ancestors shifted to a diet based on fruits, which are easier to digest, their ceca shrank. The appendix, Darwin believed, is just a shriveled up part of the cecum, which evolution hasn't entirely eliminated.

The 'Safe House' Theory of the Appendix

Some scientists now believe the appendix is not useless after all, and may help our guts recover after a gastrointestinal disease strikes.

The appendix contains a particular type of tissue associated with the lymphatic system, which carries the white blood cells needed to fight infections. In recent years, scientists have found that lymphatic tissue encourages the growth of some beneficial gut bacteria, which play an important role in human digestion and immunity.

Studies have also shown that the lining of the gut contains a biofilm, or a thin layer of microbes, mucus, and immune system molecules — and these biofilms appear to be most pronounced in the appendix.

According to the so-called "safe house" theory, the appendix protects a collection of beneficial gut bacteria when certain diseases wipe them out from elsewhere in the GI tract. Once the immune system has rid the body of the infection, the bacteria emerge from the appendix biofilm and recolonize the gut.

A review of the relevant available research published in 2016 concluded that the appendix is not a rudimentary organ but an "important part" of the immune system.

Researchers have recently found that numerous animals, including great apes, other primates, opossums, wombats, rabbits, and certain rodents all have structures similar to the appendix.

The appendix, it seems, may have independently evolved in different animals at least 32 times over the course of history, suggesting the organ does have an important function.

Appendicitis and Other Potential Health Issues

Sometimes, the appendix can become inflamed and infected, resulting in a condition called appendicitis.

Appendicitis is often the result of an abdominal infection that has spread to the tiny organ, or some kind of obstruction that has blocked the small opening of the appendix. Sources of blockage include, among other things:

• Hard pieces of stool

• Parasites or intestinal worms

• Ingested objects, including air gun pellets and pins

• Abdominal trauma

• GI tract ulcers

• Enlarged appendix lymphatic tissue

The infection or obstruction causes the bacteria in the appendix to grow out of control, and the organ can fill with pus and swell. Appendicitis causes intense abdominal pain and other GI symptoms, including vomiting and diarrhea.

Removal of the appendix (an appendectomy) is often the necessary course of action, though increasingly, antibiotics may be recommended and used to treat the infection without the need for surgical intervention — depending on the severity of the case and other health factors in the individual patient. If the problem is left untreated, the pressure in the organ will increase until the appendix ruptures, or bursts.

When the appendix bursts, it spreads its contents throughout the abdomen, potentially infecting the peritoneum, which is the silk-like membrane that lines the abdominal cavity. A peritoneum infection, called peritonitis, can then lead to sepsis, a complication that's potentially deadly if not treated aggressively.

What Is Appendicitis?

Appendicitis occurs when your appendix becomes inflamed, likely due to a blockage. It can cause symptoms like cramping or intense abdominal pain. Treatment typically involves antibiotics followed by surgery to remove your appendix.

The appendix is a small pouch attached to the intestine and is located in your lower-right abdomen. When your appendix becomes blocked, bacteria can multiply inside it. This can lead to the formation of pus and swelling, which can cause painful pressure in your abdomen. Appendicitis can also block blood flow.

If your appendix bursts, bacteria can spill into your abdominal cavity, which can be serious and sometimes fatal. If you think you may have appendicitis, it's important to speak with a doctor as soon as possible, as it requires immediate medical attention.

What is acute appendicitis vs. chronic appendicitis?

Appendicitis is almost always an acute condition, which means it begins suddenly and worsens quickly. Most of what we know about appendicitis refers to acute appendicitis, which is very common. Chronic appendicitis is a rare condition that we don't know as much about. It appears to occur when something irritates your appendix in an on-and-off sort of way over a long period, but it never gets worse.

Chronic appendicitis may go unrecognized because the symptoms don't escalate the way they do in acute appendicitis. But any type of appendicitis is serious. If you have chronic abdominal pain and you don't know what causes it, it's important to see a healthcare provider about it. Chronic appendicitis may worsen or become acute at any time. Because of this risk, healthcare providers treat it the same way.

How common is appendicitis?

Acute appendicitis is common, especially between the ages of 10 and 30. Appendicitis in children is most common during the teen years, but younger children also get it. In the U.S., about 5% of the population will get acute appendicitis in their lifetime. It's the leading cause of abdominal pain leading to emergency abdominal surgery. Chronic appendicitis occurs in approximately 1% of the population.

Causes and Risk Factors That May Predispose You to Appendicitis

Causes

In the U.S., 1 in 20 people will get appendicitis at some point in their lives. Although it can strike at any age, appendicitis is rare in children younger than 2. It's most likely to affect people between the ages of 10 and 30 and people who were assigned male at birth. If appendicitis runs in your family, you might also be more likely to get it at some point. It's not a condition that's passed down, but some genetic factors could put you at a higher risk.

Appendicitis happens when the appendix gets blocked, often by poop, a foreign body (something inside you that isn't supposed to be there), or cancer. Blockage may also result from infection since the appendix can swell in response to any infection in the body.

In many cases, the exact cause of appendicitis is unknown. Experts believe it develops when part of the appendix becomes obstructed or blocked.

Many things can potentially block your appendix, including:

- a buildup of hardened stool

- enlarged lymphoid follicles

- intestinal worms

- traumatic injury

- tumors

Appendicitis can affect anyone. However, some people may be more likely to develop this condition than others. Risk factors for appendicitis include:

- **Age**: Appendicitis most often affects teenagers and people in their 20s, but it can occur at any age.

- **Sex**: Appendicitis is more common in males than females.

- **Family history**: People who have a family history of appendicitis are at heightened risk of developing it.

Appendicitis in pregnancy

Acute appendicitis is the most common non-obstetric emergency requiring surgery during pregnancy.

The symptoms of appendicitis may be mistaken for routine discomfort from pregnancy. Pregnancy may also cause your appendix to shift upward in your abdomen, which can affect the location of appendicitis-related pain. This can make it harder to diagnose.

Delayed diagnosis and treatment may increase your risk of complications, including miscarriage.

What causes chronic appendicitis?

The theory of chronic appendicitis is that something causes mild inflammation on and off for a long time. It might be a chronic condition like inflammatory bowel disease or mild bacterial overgrowth. Or it might be an obstruction that moves in and out of the opening to your appendix. Chronic inflammation can lead to lymphoid hyperplasia or even scar tissue in your appendix if it lasts a very long time.

Is appendicitis genetic?

Having a family history of appendicitis does appear to raise your risk of developing it, though it's not clear why. Appendicitis itself is not inherited, but genetics might be involved in some of its causes.

Can stress cause appendicitis?

It's not likely. However, severe physiological stress from critical illness can cause bowel ischemia, a temporary reduction of blood flow to your intestines. Ischemic colitis may rarely affect your appendix.

Can food cause appendicitis?

There have been rare reports of an undigested seed or nut getting stuck in the opening to the appendix and causing inflammation. In general, though, eating more fiber reduces your risk of appendicitis.

Risk factors

Risk factors for appendicitis include:

- Age. Anyone can develop appendicitis, but it most often happens in people between the ages of 10 and 30.

- Your sex. Men have a slightly higher risk of appendicitis than do women.

Do I Have Appendicitis? Symptoms to Check for and Diagnostic Evaluations

The classic symptoms of appendicitis include:

- Pain in your lower right belly or pain near your navel that moves lower. This is usually the first sign. The appendix pain location might be different for some people, depending on where your appendix is. If it's behind your colon, for example, you may feel pain near your pelvis. If you're pregnant, the pain might start higher up, as the appendix can move during pregnancy.

- Loss of appetite

- Nausea and vomiting soon after belly pain begins

- Swollen belly

- Fever of 99-102 F

- Inability to pass gas

Other less common symptoms of appendicitis include:

- Dull or sharp pain anywhere in your upper or lower belly, back, or rear end

- Painful or difficult peeing

- Vomiting before your belly pain starts

- Severe cramps

- Constipation or diarrhea with gas

Atypical signs of appendicitis during pregnancy include:

- Acid reflux and/or indigestion

- Pelvic pain

- Pain beneath your rib cage

- Pain when urinating

If you have any of these symptoms, see a doctor right away. Acute appendicitis comes on suddenly and develops quickly over 24 hours. Timely diagnosis and treatment are important. Don't eat, drink, or use any pain remedies, antacids, laxatives, or heating pads.

How can I check for appendicitis at home?

If you suspect appendicitis, you should always have a healthcare provider check for it. But if you're looking for a sign, there are a few that healthcare providers use to check for appendicitis. Pain location can be a helpful clue, especially if it begins around your navel and then moves to your lower right abdomen in the typical fashion. But some people feel the pain elsewhere. Providers may look for:

- **McBurney's sign**. McBurney's point is the most typical location of the appendix, and tenderness there is the first thing healthcare providers check for in a physical exam. They find it by drawing a line from your ASIS (a bony projection near your hip) to your belly button and measuring the distance. The point is about two inches along the line, or one-third of the distance.

- **Blumberg's sign**. Pressure applied to the sore area feels worse when it's released (also known as rebound tenderness).

- **Dunphy's sign**. Coughing makes the pain worse.

- **Rovsing's sign**. Pressure on your lower left side produces pain on your lower right side.

- **Psoas sign.** If your appendix is behind your colon rather than in front, appendicitis might irritate your psoas muscle. You might find yourself flexing your right hip to shorten the muscle, which relieves pain. A healthcare provider might try extending your right hip or rotating it outward. If this hurts, it's called the psoas sign. If rotating it inward hurts, it's called the obturator sign.

What other conditions might be confused with appendicitis?

Symptoms of appendicitis can resemble many other conditions. This is especially true for women and people assigned female at birth (AFAB). Your lower abdomen lies close to your pelvic cavity, and conditions affecting your pelvic organs may feel very similar to appendicitis. These organs include your urinary system and female reproductive system. Other lower abdominal organs may also be involved.

Some common conditions that might be easily confused with appendicitis include:

- Pelvic inflammatory disease.

- Endometriosis.

- Ovarian cyst.

- Kidney stone.

- Urinary tract infection.

- Pancreatitis.

- Inflammatory bowel disease.

- Diverticulitis of the colon.

- Gastroenteritis.

- Intestinal obstruction.

How is appendicitis diagnosed?

If a doctor suspects you might have appendicitis, they will begin by talking with you about your symptoms and medical history. They'll then perform a physical exam to check for tenderness in the lower right part of your abdomen and swelling or rigidity.

There's no single test available to diagnose appendicitis.

Depending on the results of your physical exam, a doctor may order 1 or more of the following tests to check for signs of appendicitis:

Blood tests

To check for signs of infection, a doctor may order a complete blood count (CBC).

They may also order a C-reactive protein test to determine whether there are other causes of abdominal inflammation, such as an autoimmune disorder.

Urine tests

Appendicitis can display similar symptoms to a urinary tract infection (UTI) or kidney stones. A doctor will typically run a urine test to rule out these conditions.

Pregnancy test

Ectopic pregnancy can be mistaken for appendicitis. It happens when a fertilized egg implants itself in a fallopian tube, rather than the uterus. This can be a medical emergency.

If a doctor suspects you might have an ectopic pregnancy, they may perform a pregnancy test. To conduct this test, they will collect a sample of your urine or blood. They may also use a transvaginal ultrasound to learn where the fertilized egg has implanted.

Depending on the location of the ectopic pregnancy, a doctor may suggest treating the condition using medication or surgery.

Abdominal imaging tests

To check for inflammation of your appendix, a doctor may order imaging tests of your abdomen.

It can also help doctors identify other potential causes of your symptoms, such as:

- abdominal abscess

- fecal impaction

- inflammatory bowel disease (IBD)

In some cases, you may be asked to stop eating food for a short period before your test. A doctor can help you learn more about preparing for your test.

Complications

Appendicitis can cause serious complications if your appendix ruptures, as this cause fecal matter and bacteria to spill into your abdominal cavity. A ruptured appendix can lead to painful and potentially life-threatening infections.

This includes:

- **Peritonitis**: When the appendix bursts and bacteria spill into your abdominal cavity, the lining can become infected and inflamed. This is known as peritonitis. It can be very serious and even fatal. Treatment includes antibiotics and surgery to remove the appendix.

• **Abscesses**: An abscess is a painful pocket of pus that forms around a burst appendix. These white blood cells are your body's way of fighting the infection. The infection must be treated with antibiotics, and the abscess will need to be drained.

• **Sepsis**: In rare cases, bacteria from a ruptured abscess may travel through your bloodstream to other parts of your body. Sepsis is a medical emergency. If you suspect you have sepsis, call 911 immediately.

• **Ileus**. In some cases, the inflammation of the appendix can trigger ileus, which is when your intestines stop contracting and food can't move through your digestive system. It's temporary but might make you feel constipated, bloated, and gassy.

- **Fistula.** While rare, it's also possible for a fistula to form after an appendectomy. A fistula is a passage between two body parts that shouldn't be there. In the case of appendicitis, a fistula can form involving the intestines. Fistulas require surgery to fix.

To prevent or manage complications, a doctor may prescribe antibiotics, surgery, or other treatments. In some cases, you might develop side effects or complications from the treatment.

However, the risks associated with antibiotics and surgery are far less common and usually less serious than the potential complications of untreated appendicitis.

Treatment and Prevention Strategies for Managing Appendicitis

The NIDDK states that a doctor will prescribe antibiotics for anyone with appendicitis.

In some cases, this is enough to treat appendicitis, and surgery will not be necessary. In most cases, however, a surgeon must remove the appendix. This is called an appendectomy.

According to a 2023 review and meta-analysis, although the cure rate is lower than with surgery, treatment with antibiotics may be an option for those with uncomplicated acute appendicitis who do not wish to have surgery.

There are two methods for removing the appendix, which include:

Laparoscopy

This is the most common type of appendectomy because of its quick recovery time. During surgery, a doctor will use a tube to inflate your abdomen with gas so that they can see your appendix better. They will remove your appendix through a 4-inch-long cut or with a device called a laparoscope (a thin telescope-like tool that lets them see inside your belly). If you have peritonitis, the surgeon will also clean out your belly and drain the pus. The surgeon will close the cut with either dissolvable or regular stitches. If you get regular stitches, you'll need to visit your doctor 7-10 days after surgery to have them removed. You should be able to leave the hospital within 24 hours if there aren't any complications.

Open surgery

If your appendix has already burst, or if you've had open abdominal surgery in the past, your doctor will make a larger cut in the lower right side of your belly. Once the abdominal area is open, the surgeon will tie off your appendix with stitches and remove it. If your appendix has burst, your abdomen will be washed out with salt water. The cut will be closed with stitches and a small tube may be inserted to drain any extra fluids. If you have peritonitis, your doctor may have to make a cut along the middle of your abdomen. It could take up to 1 week before you're able to leave the hospital.

After surgery, you may be given pain relievers through an IV. You can drink liquids within a few hours and slowly start to eat more solid foods. After 12 hours, you should be able to get up and move around. It's normal to have some pain and bruising around the cut. If you had a laparoscopy, you might also have pain in your shoulder or feel bloated from the gas that was pumped into your belly. You can take over-the-counter painkillers to help. It's important to keep the cut clean and dry while it heals.

To help with your recovery, limit your activity for 3-5 days after a laparoscopy and 10-14 days after open surgery. If you need to cough, you can support your abdomen by placing a pillow over it and applying pressure. Slowly increase your activity as you feel up for it, starting with short walks, but also rest when you need to. You should be able to go back to your normal routine in 2-3 weeks, but if you had open surgery, avoid strenuous activities for 4-6 weeks.

After an appendectomy, call your doctor if you have:

- Uncontrolled vomiting

- Increased belly pain

- Dizziness/feelings of faintness

- Blood in your vomit or pee

- Increased pain and redness where your doctor cut into your belly

- Fever

- Pus in the wound

Recovery time for appendicitis

According to the United Kingdom's National Health Service (NHS), a person who has had laparoscopic surgery can go home after 24 hours.

If open surgery was necessary, they may have to stay in the hospital for up to a week.

For the first few days, a person may experience some constipation, pain, and bruising.

There may also be pain at the tip of the shoulder. During the surgery, the surgeon pumps gas into the abdomen. This can stimulate the phrenic nerve at the diaphragm, causing referred pain. Referred pain occurs at a location other than where the real source of pain exists.

Over-the-counter (OTC) pain relievers may help with postsurgical pain.

After a couple of weeks, a person should be able to resume their usual activities. However, they may need to avoid strenuous activity for 4 to 6 weeks.

The doctor will advise about how much activity is suitable at each stage of recovery.

If there are signs of infection, it is important to contact the doctor.

Signs of infection include:

- worsening pain and swelling

- repeated vomiting

- high temperature

- the site of the operation is hot to touch

- the site of the operation has pus or other discharge

Prevention

There's no sure way to prevent appendicitis. But you might be able to lower your risk of developing it by eating a fiber-rich diet.

Foods high in fiber include:

- fruits

- vegetables

- lentils, split peas, beans, and other legumes

- oatmeal, brown rice, whole wheat, and other whole grains

A doctor may also suggest you take a fiber supplement.

Add fiber by:

- sprinkling oat bran or wheat germ over breakfast cereals, yogurt, and salads

- cooking or baking with whole-wheat flour whenever possible

- swapping white rice for brown rice

- adding kidney beans or other legumes to salads

- eating fresh fruit for dessert

2
APPENDICITIS PRE-SURGERY DIET

Diet plays an important role in the recovery process after appendicitis surgery. A proper diet can help ensure a safe and quick recovery. Here are some tips for what to eat and avoid after appendicitis surgery:

- **Eat protein**: Protein is important for tissue repair and building muscles. Lean proteins like chicken, fish, tofu, and legumes are gentle on the digestive system.

- **Eat fiber**: A high-fiber diet can help with constipation and make it easier to go to the bathroom without straining your abdominal muscles. Whole grains, fruits, and vegetables are all good sources of fiber.

- **Eat small meals**: Smaller meals are easier to digest and cause less stomach stretching, which can put stress on your healing gut.

- **Drink enough water**: Hydration helps with healing and keeps the digestive system working properly. You should aim to drink at least eight glasses of water a day.

- **Avoid high-fat foods**: High-fat foods are difficult to digest and should be avoided.

- **Avoid spicy foods**: Spicy foods can irritate the gastrointestinal tract and increase pain and inflammation.

- **Avoid caffeinated beverages**: Caffeine can stimulate the digestive system and cause discomfort.

Avoid refined or synthetic sugar: Refined or synthetic sugar can trigger diarrhea and aggravate symptoms.

Foods to Avoid to Prevent Worsening Symptoms

What should you not eat or drink after appendicitis surgery?

There are some foods you should avoid after having your appendix removed, even if you get the all clear to go back to your regular diet.

Try to avoid high-fat and fried foods. They can cause indigestion, nausea, and diarrhea. After appendicitis surgery, try to limit or avoid foods like:

Spicy Foods

- **Reason to Avoid:** Spicy foods can irritate the gastrointestinal tract, leading to increased pain and inflammation, potentially slowing down the healing process.

- **Examples:** Hot peppers, spicy sauces, and foods seasoned with chili powder should be approached with caution during the recovery period.

Fatty and Fried Foods

- **Reason to Avoid:** High-fat foods are difficult to digest and can slow down the recovery process by straining the digestive system, potentially leading to symptoms like indigestion, bloating, and nausea, which can be particularly uncomfortable post-surgery.

- **Examples:** Fried chicken, French fries, burgers, and fatty cuts of meat. Fast foods and deep-fried snacks should be avoided to reduce the risk of digestive distress and support smoother recovery.

Dairy Products

- **Reason to Avoid:** Some people become temporarily lactose intolerant after abdominal surgery, leading to bloating, gas, and diarrhea. The lactose in dairy products can ferment in the gut, causing discomfort and potentially worsening post-surgical symptoms.

- **Examples:** Milk, cheese, yogurt, and cream-based products. If dairy is necessary, lactose-free options or plant-based alternatives like almond milk or coconut yogurt can be considered.

Carbonated Beverages

- **Reason to Avoid:** Carbonated drinks can cause gas and bloating, which are uncomfortable and potentially harmful after surgery.

- **Examples:** Soda and carbonated energy drinks. Sticking to still water and non-carbonated beverages can help maintain hydration without the added discomfort of gas.

Caffeinated Beverages

- **Reason to Avoid:** Caffeine can cause dehydration and may irritate the digestive tract, prolonging recovery. It can also increase acid production in the stomach, leading to further irritation and discomfort.

- **Examples:** Coffee, tea, and energy drinks. Herbal teas and decaffeinated beverages are better alternatives during the recovery period to ensure hydration and minimize irritation.

Are there any permanent dietary changes you should make after appendicitis surgery?

No. You don't need to permanently change your diet if you've had your appendix removed.

The appendix is part of the intestine, so it's natural to assume that your intestines won't work the same without it. But according to Dr. Emilia Genova, a general surgeon with Hartford Healthcare, the appendix doesn't help with digestion. So, there isn't any need to make long-term dietary changes after having your appendix removed.

But again, it depends on the circumstances surrounding your appendectomy. Dr. Genova said, "Sometimes, if the patients have been ill, have had a perforation of the appendix, or needed a more extensive surgery — such as bowel resection — diet changes may be indicated." But even in these cases, Dr. Genova noted that these changes are usually only temporary and short term.

When should you contact your healthcare provider after appendicitis surgery?

It's normal to have some mild abdominal discomfort and nausea after appendicitis surgery. If you had laparoscopic surgery, you might also notice some shoulder or neck pain from the gas used to inflate your abdomen during surgery. These symptoms will improve with time.

But some symptoms are more concerning. You should contact your surgical team right away if:

- Your pain isn't getting better after 2 or 3 days

- Your pain is getting worse at any time after surgery

- You're unable to keep food or liquids down

- You haven't had a bowel movement within 48 hours after surgery

- You develop a fever

- You notice redness, discharge, swelling, or pain around your incision (stitches)

Pre-Surgery Hydration Tips

Staying properly hydrated before appendix surgery is crucial for maintaining overall health and preparing your body for the procedure. Here are some practical tips to ensure adequate hydration:

1. Prioritize Water Intake

- Water should be your primary source of hydration leading up to the surgery. Aim for at least 8-10 glasses of water daily, unless otherwise directed by your doctor.

- Sip water consistently throughout the day rather than drinking large amounts at once to avoid overloading your system.

2. Incorporate Electrolytes

- If allowed, include electrolyte-rich fluids like coconut water, oral rehydration solutions, or electrolyte-infused drinks to maintain a healthy balance of minerals like sodium, potassium, and magnesium.

- Avoid sugary sports drinks, as they can be counterproductive and may irritate your stomach.

3. Limit Diuretics

- Cut back on beverages that act as diuretics, such as coffee, tea, or alcohol, as they can lead to dehydration.

- Opt for herbal teas or caffeine-free options if you crave a warm drink.

4. Follow Fasting Guidelines

- If your doctor has instructed you to fast before surgery, follow their guidelines strictly. Typically, clear fluids may be allowed up to a certain point before surgery.

- Confirm with your healthcare provider how long you can consume clear fluids before the procedure.

5. Choose Clear Liquids When Necessary

- If on a clear liquid diet before surgery, include broths, clear juices (apple or white grape), and plain water to stay hydrated.

- Avoid liquids with pulp, carbonation, or dairy, as these may upset your stomach or interfere with pre-surgery preparations.

6. Stay Mindful of Symptoms

- Pay attention to signs of dehydration, such as dark urine, fatigue, or dizziness, and increase your fluid intake accordingly.

- If you feel nauseous or have trouble drinking fluids, inform your healthcare provider for additional guidance.

Proper hydration not only supports your body during surgery but also aids in recovery by maintaining optimal circulation, reducing the risk of complications, and ensuring better overall health. Always consult your medical team for specific hydration instructions tailored to your condition.

Role of Low-Fiber Foods in Reducing Inflammation

Fiber is the part of fruits, vegetables and grains not digested by your body. A low-fiber diet limits these foods in the diet. As a result, there is less undigested material moving through the large intestine, and stools are less bulky.

A low-fiber diet may be recommended for a number of conditions or situations. It is sometimes called a restricted-fiber diet.

Purpose

Reasons your health care provider may prescribe a low-fiber diet include:

- You have narrowing of the bowel. This may be due to a tumor or an inflammatory disease, such as Crohn's disease and ulcerative colitis.

- You have had bowel surgery.

- You are having treatment that damages or irritates your digestive system. For example, radiation can cause irritation.

Low-fiber diets are usually temporary. You can usually start to add more fiber back into your diet after a short amount of time.

Diet details

A low-fiber diet limits the types of vegetables, fruits and grains that you can eat. Some of the foods that are allowed on a low-fiber diet include milk, cheese, yogurt, meat, fish and eggs. People who are lactose intolerant should avoid milk and dairy products if they cause stomach pain or diarrhea.

The ability to digest food varies from person to person. A health care provider may recommend a diet that is more or less limited depending on the reasons it is being used.

If you're eating a low-fiber diet, be sure to read food labels. Foods you might not expect can have added fiber. For example, yogurt, ice cream, cereal and even some drinks may have fiber. Look for foods that have no more than 1 to 2 grams of fiber in one serving.

Avoid these foods and products made with them:

- Nuts, seeds, dried fruit and coconut.

- Whole grains, popcorn, wheat germ and bran.

- Brown rice, wild rice, oatmeal, granola, shredded wheat, quinoa, bulgur and barley.

- Dried beans, baked beans, lima beans, peas and lentils.

- Chunky peanut butter.

- Fruits and vegetables except those noted below.

Choose these foods:

- Tender meat, fish and poultry, ham, bacon, shellfish, and lunch meat.

- Eggs, tofu and creamy peanut butter.

- Dairy products if tolerated.

- White rice and pasta.

- Baked goods made with refined wheat or rye flour, such as bread, biscuits, pancakes, waffles, bagels, saltines and graham crackers.

- Hot and cold cereals that have less than 2 grams of dietary fiber in a single serving. Cereals made with rice cereals often have very little fiber.

- Canned or well-cooked potatoes, carrots and green beans.

- Plain tomato sauce.

- Vegetable and fruit juices.

- Bananas, melons, applesauce and canned peaches (no skin).

- Butter, margarine, oils and salad dressings without seeds.

A typical menu might look like this:

Breakfast

- Cornflakes with milk.
- White toast, creamy peanut butter, jelly.
- Fruit juice.
- Coffee.

Midmorning snack

- Yogurt without seeds.
- Water or other beverage.

Noon meal

- Turkey sandwich on white bread with mayonnaise.

- Tomato soup.

- Canned peaches.

- Milk or other beverage.

Afternoon snack

- Cheese slices.

- Saltine crackers.

- Water or other beverage.

Evening meal

- Baked fish.

- Mashed potatoes with butter.

- Cooked carrots.

- Applesauce.

- Milk or other beverage.

Prepare all foods so that they're tender. Good cooking methods include simmering, poaching, stewing, steaming and braising. Baking or microwaving in a covered dish is another option.

You may have fewer bowel movements and smaller stools on a low-fiber diet. To avoid constipation, you may need to drink extra fluids. Drink plenty of water unless your health care provider tells you otherwise.

Results

Eating a low-fiber diet will limit your bowel movements. It may help reduce diarrhea or other symptoms, such as stomach pain. After a short time, you may be able to slowly introduce fiber into your diet again.

Risks

Because a low-fiber diet limits what you can eat, it can be difficult to meet your nutritional needs. You should follow a low-fiber diet only as long as directed by your health care provider.

If you must continue eating this diet for a longer time, consult a registered dietitian. A dietitian can help make sure you are meeting all of your nutritional needs.

3

POST-SURGERY DIET: HEALING AND RECOVERY

You've just had surgery for appendicitis — this surgery is called an appendectomy. You're hungry, and your body needs nourishment to help you heal. While you might feel ready to eat, you can't go right back to your usual diet. Instead, you have to take a stepwise approach to give your bowels time to recover.

When can you eat after appendicitis surgery?

Most people are able to start eating within a few hours after their appendicitis surgery.

You can usually start sipping water as soon as you wake up and your anesthesia wears off after surgery. Once your surgical team examines you, they'll likely give you the "all clear" to drink other clear liquids such as:

- Broth

- Jell-O

- Popsicles

- Clear sodas (like sprite or ginger ale)

- Fruit juices without pulp (like apple or cranberry juice)

If you're able to consume these clear liquids without any trouble for about a day, your surgical team will give you the "OK" to start solid foods. Most people are able to eat solid food about 24 hours after appendicitis surgery.

Once you are cleared to eat solid foods, it's best to start with bland and low-fat foods such as:

- Well-cooked, soft cereals

- Mashed potatoes

- Plain toast

- Plain crackers

- Plain pasta

- Rice

- Cottage cheese

- Pudding

- Low-fat yogurt

- Ripe bananas

You'll want to try small meals at first. Smaller meals are easier for your body to digest. Eating six to eight small meals a day can be gentler on your healing gut than three regular-sized meals. Plus, smaller meals cause less stomach stretching (distension). Stretching can put stress on your healing gut and stitches, leading to pain.

After 1 to 2 days, try to incorporate high-fiber foods like whole grains, fruits, and vegetables into your diet. And make sure to drink enough water. These two changes can help you fight off the constipation that often happens after surgery.

People develop constipation after surgery for several reasons:

- **Pain medications:** Most people need to take pain medications for a few days after having their appendix removed. Opioid pain medications help with pain control, but they also cause constipation.

- **Slow gut movement:** You'll want to take it easy after surgery. But being less active can also slow down your gut. And your gut is also trying to recover from both appendicitis and surgery. This means it may not work as well as it usually does. These two things will slow down your gut, increasing your risk of developing constipation.

A high-fiber diet will make it easy to go to the bathroom without straining the abdominal muscles.

- Have a balanced diet- Once you've started eating solid meals, you'll want to make sure you're receiving enough nutrients from all food categories. You are more likely to lose energy, feel weak, and not recover correctly if you restrict yourself too much. Protein, whole grains, veggies, and fruits are all necessary.

- Add colorful fresh fruits to your diet- Fresh fruits and vegetables are high in fiber and minerals. These components are critical for healing during your post-surgery recovery and for maintaining your immune system's health. While fresh foods are considered healthier, frozen or tinned foods are also acceptable.

- Whole grains are a must - as per the laparoscopic appendicectomy doctor in

Jayanagar, Whole grains are high in vitamins and minerals, as well as fiber.

- So, wherever feasible, pick whole-grain bread and cereals over-processed white ones.

Breakfast is an excellent time to incorporate healthy grains and fiber into your diet. For your morning meal, choose oatmeal or similar whole-grain cereal, whole wheat bread, and fresh fruit.

- Zinc-rich foods - Zinc deficiency in the diet might interfere with the body's natural healing mechanism. Oysters, egg yolks, plant seeds, peanuts, and milk products are among the best sources of this essential vitamin.

- Focus on low-fat dairy products- Nature has given us a wonderful healing meal neatly packaged in a shell. For good reason, eggs are a customary first meal served to invalids and recuperating patients.

Can appendix patients eat eggs?

One egg contains the following nutrients:

- The protein content of 6 grams

- A, E, and K vitamins

- Vitamins of the B complex (including B12)

- Riboflavin

- The mineral folic acid

- iron

- Calcium a

- zinc

All of the nutrients we've already mentioned as being essential for a rapid recovery. The best aspect is that eggs are simple to cook and serve.

Staying Hydrated for Digestive Wellness

Among its many functions in the body, water is critical to healthy digestion by supporting the process from start to finish.

If you're like many people, healthy digestion might be more top of mind than it used to be. Part of this renewed interest in digestive health may have to do with an abundance of emerging science on the importance of maintaining a healthy "gut microbiome" – the collection of bacteria that inhabits the digestive tract and which affects the health of many systems in the body.

And so, to keep your digestive system healthy and happy, you may be aware of the importance of taking in probiotics (the "good" bacteria) as well as prebiotics (such as certain forms of fiber that serve as "food" for the probiotics) and adequate fiber, which helps move waste through your system and promotes regularity.

But there's something much simpler and more basic to keeping your digestive system running smoothly: water. Water is involved in literally every step of the digestive process, which is just another reason why staying adequately hydrated is so critically important to your health.

How Does Water Aid Digestion?

Starting at the very beginning of the digestive process, water is a major component of your saliva.

Saliva serves several functions:

- It helps to moisten your food, which makes it easier to chew and swallow.

- It is also a vehicle for enzymes that begin the process of chemically breaking down the fats and carbohydrates as you chew.

As the food passes into your stomach, watery gastric juices are released. These juices also contain enzymes, which begin to break the proteins and carbohydrates in the foods you eat into smaller parts, preparing them for their trip to the small intestine, where much of your food's digestion occurs. Water is also needed to produce the mucus that coats the inside of your stomach, which protects it from highly acidic digestive juices.

By the way, there's no truth to the myth that drinking water with meals will dilute the digestive juices so much that they can't do their job. Adequate fluid with meals helps promote the process.

How Water Supports a Healthy Bowel

As the food moves through the small intestine, there's a lot of digestive activity that water facilitates:

• More watery secretions are shot into the small intestine from the intestinal lining itself as well as from the pancreas and liver.

• Enzymes work to speed up chemical processes and help prepare for the absorption of the end products of digestion: amino acids from proteins, fatty acids from fats and individual sugar molecules from the carbohydrates you eat.

• Most nutrient absorption takes place here in the small bowel, and then digested nutrients pass to the watery environment of your bloodstream.

As the digestive process continues in the large bowel, water is critically important, too:

• The soluble fibers that you eat (from foods like oats, beans and barley) dissolve in water, allowing them to swell and add bulk.

• The insoluble fiber that you eat (from foods like whole grains and most vegetables) tends to trap and attract water rather than absorb it, which helps promote regular bowel movements.

The lower bowel is also where your body takes up most of the minerals that you eat, and the watery environment there facilitates their absorption.

There's no question that healthy digestion relies on adequate fiber (and probiotics are a good idea, too). Exercise is also important – when you move your skeletal muscles during exercise, you're stimulating the smooth muscles of your digestive tract at the same time, which helps promote regularity. But don't forget the simplest and most basic thing of all – make sure to take in plenty of fluids every day to keep your system running smoothly.

Managing Digestive Sensitivities Post-Surgery

If you've recently undergone surgery, you may be experiencing digestive issues as part of your recovery process. Digestive problems such as bloating, constipation, and diarrhea after surgery are common and can be uncomfortable. However, there are steps you can take to manage and alleviate these post-surgery digestive issues.

Eat a Balanced Diet

Post-surgery rehabilitation includes paying attention to your diet. Consuming a balanced diet is essential for maintaining a healthy digestive system. Incorporate a variety of fruits, vegetables, whole grains, and lean proteins into your meals.

These nutrient-rich foods provide the necessary nutrients and fiber needed for proper digestion.

Avoid foods that are difficult to digest, such as fried, greasy, and processed foods. These types of foods can exacerbate digestive issues and slow down the digestion process. Opt for lighter, easier-to-digest foods like steamed vegetables, baked chicken, and whole grains.

Stay Hydrated

Proper hydration is crucial for a healthy digestive system. Drinking enough water helps soften stool and prevents constipation. Aim to drink at least 8 glasses of water per day, or more if recommended by your healthcare provider. Avoid excessive consumption of caffeinated and sugary beverages as they can dehydrate your body and worsen digestive issues.

Chew Your Food Slowly

Take the time to chew your food properly and slowly. Chewing thoroughly breaks down the food into smaller, more easily digestible pieces. This allows the digestive enzymes in your saliva to begin breaking down carbohydrates and proteins before they reach your stomach. Eating too quickly can lead to indigestion and contribute to bloating and discomfort.

Avoid Straws and Carbonated Beverages

Using straws and consuming carbonated beverages can introduce excess air into your digestive system, leading to bloating and gas. Therefore, it's best to avoid using straws and limit your intake of carbonated drinks until your digestive system has fully recovered.

Exercise Regularly

Regular physical activity can help stimulate your digestive system and promote healthy bowel movements. Engage in light exercise such as walking or gentle stretching, as recommended by your healthcare provider. However, avoid strenuous activities that could put strain on your body and impede the healing process.

Avoid Smoking and Alcohol

Both smoking and excessive alcohol consumption can negatively impact your digestive system. Smoking can weaken the muscles of the digestive tract, leading to slower digestion and increased risk of acid reflux. Alcohol can irritate the stomach lining and contribute to inflammation. It's best to avoid smoking and limit alcohol intake to promote a healthy digestive system.

Manage Stress

Stress can have various effects on the body, including digestive issues. Research shows that stress can alter gut function and exacerbate digestive symptoms. Use relaxation techniques such as deep breathing exercises, meditation, or yoga to manage stress levels. Additionally, consider engaging in activities that bring you joy and help you unwind.

Consider Probiotics

Probiotics are beneficial bacteria that can promote a healthy gut. They can help restore the balance of bacteria in your digestive system, improving digestion and reducing symptoms such as bloating and diarrhea. Talk to your healthcare provider about whether taking a probiotic supplement is appropriate for you post-surgery.

Follow Your Doctor's Recommendations

Every individual's post-surgery recovery is unique, so it's important to follow your doctor's specific recommendations regarding diet, activity level, and any prescribed medications. Your healthcare provider will provide guidance tailored to your specific needs.

Managing post-surgery digestive issues requires patience and a proactive approach. By incorporating these tips into your daily routine, you can help alleviate digestive discomfort and support a healthy recovery.

Constipation After Surgery: Tips for Relief

Constipation is a side effect of surgery that you may not have expected. It's common, even if your bowel movements were regular before your operation.

It can happen for many reasons, including:

Side effects from meds: The anesthesia you get before surgery and the prescriptions you fill afterward (including pain medications, diuretics, and muscle relaxants) could be the problem.

Your diet changed: Your doctor might have told you not to eat or drink in the hours leading up to the surgery, or put you on a restrictive diet after the operation. The combination of too little fluid and food can affect your bowel movements, making you more likely to become constipated.

You can't exercise yet: If you need to stay in a hospital bed or can't work out for a while as you recover, that lack of movement can slow down your digestion and make it harder to pass stool. Inactivity is a common cause of constipation.

The problem may not last long, and you can take steps to get your system moving again.

What Helps

Drink more. Dehydration makes constipation more likely. Water helps break down the food in your stomach, assisting with digestion. Research shows that downing at least four glasses of water per day can help prevent constipation.

Avoid caffeine. It's dehydrating, which can make matters worse. So, you may need to halt the coffee, tea, and caffeinated soda (plus chocolate) for now.

Add fiber. It helps you pass stools and stay regular. Most adults should get between 22 and 34 grams of fiber per day. Foods such as bran, beans, apples, pears, prunes, squash, sweet potatoes, spinach, and collard greens are good sources of fiber. If you don't have much of an appetite after surgery, try a smoothie made with fruits and vegetables.

Get moving. As soon as your doctor says it's OK, get up and move around as much as possible. Even a short walk down the hospital hallway will help. Exercise helps move digested food through your intestines and signals your body that it's time for a bowel movement.

Consider medications. Your doctor may recommend stool softeners, which make stool easier to pass, or laxatives, which pull water into your intestines and help stool move along the intestinal tract.

If laxatives and stool softeners don't do the trick, suppositories may help. You insert them into your rectum to soften stool and trigger your intestinal muscles to squeeze, making it easier to pass stool. Both prescription and over-the-counter options are available.

Ask about dietary supplements. Some, including fiber, kefir, and carnitine, may help ease constipation. Other supplements, such as iron, can make constipation worse. Talk to your doctor before you start to take any dietary supplements, to make sure they're OK for you.

4
APPENDICITIS DIET RECIPES YOU MUST TRY

BREAKFAST RECIPES TO START YOUR DAY RIGHT

Creamy cherry smoothie (low Fiber)

Ingredients

- 1/4 ripe avocado

- 100 ml dark cherry juice

- 1 teaspoon hulled tahini

- 1 teaspoon lecithin granules

- 150 ml unsweetened oat milk

- 1 tablespoon coconut crème

- 1 Maraschino cherry (optional to serve)

Instructions

Add all ingredients and blend until smooth.

Serve with a split maraschino cherry on the side of the glass.

Aloo masala (Low Fiber)

Ingredients

- 4 large carrots (peeled & chopped into chunks)

- 500 grams large white peeled potato (chopped into chunks)

- 100 grams baby spinach

- 1/4 cup smooth cashew butter

- 1 teaspoon powdered garlic

- 1 bunch of coriander leaves (stalks removed, washed and roughly chopped)

- 1 lemon cut into eight pieces

- 1 teaspoon ground cumin

- 2 teaspoons garam masala

- 1 tablespoon brown sugar

- 1 cup vegetable stock

- 2 tablespoons raisins (can use 1/2 peeled apple chopped into small pieces for ostomates) - may not be suitable for ostomates

- salt and pepper grind to taste

- olive oil to cook with

Instructions

In a large heavy bottomed pan heat the olive oil and add onion and garlic sauté for one minute.

Add the potatoes, carrot, garam masala and cumin and stir for 2-3 minutes until you can smell the spices.

Add some salt and pepper and stir.

Add stock, brown sugar, raisins (or apple chunks) and simmer for 10 – 12 minutes until potatoes are soft.

Add cashew nut butter and blend through, baby spinach and coriander, cook for another two to three minutes.

Remove from the stove and squeeze half of the fresh lemon into the stew.

Serve with basmati rice and the other slices of lemon.

Eggy devils (Low Fiber)

Ingredients

- 3 tablespoons whole egg organic mayonnaise

- 6 free range eggs

- Pinch of turmeric powder

- Pinch of mustard powder

- Salt and pepper to taste

- Paprika to dust eggs with

- Packet of water crackers

Instructions

Add eggs to a saucepan, cover with water and heat. Once boiling, let the eggs cook for 4½ minutes.

Remove from heat and place the eggs into cold water for one minute then carefully peel and slice them in half lengthwise.

Gently scoop out the yolks into a bowl and mash with the mayonnaise, turmeric, mustard and salt and pepper to taste.

Cut a little slice off the rounded bottom of the egg white halves so they sit firmly on the plate or cracker without wobbling, then pipe or spoon the yolk mix back into the white egg halves.

Dust the tops lightly with paprika and serve.

Basil zoodle frittata (Low Fiber)

Ingredients

- 1/2 cup breadcrumbs
- 1 teaspoon powdered garlic
- 1/4 cup chopped fine chives
- 2 zucchinis (spiralised)
- 6 free range eggs
- 1/2 cup cottage cheese
- pinch of salt

- 1 tablespoon Cobram Estate® extra-virgin olive oil (full flavoured three drop – for a lighter taste use one or two drop variety)

- 1/4 cup torn basil leaves

Instructions

Heat oven to 180C.

Press breadcrumbs down in the base of a pie dish.

Place in oven for 10 minutes or until golden – press down again.

Lightly blanch zucchini in boiled water add salt and drain extremely well on paper towel.

In a bowl add zucchini, olive oil, chives, cottage cheese, garlic powder and bay leaves, mix through so **Ingredients** are evenly distributed.

Place in the pie dish and flatten down.

Beat eggs and pour over the top.

Bake for 20-30 minutes until golden on top and the frittata bounces back on touch.

Serve with wilted baby spinach (low Fiber) and crusty white roll.

Eastern baked eggs (*Low Fiber*)

Ingredients

- 100 grams (drained) tinned/jar red pepper (chopped finely)

- 800 grams (2 tins) diced cooked tomatoes blended (ostomates will need to strain tomatoes to remove pips)

- 2 tablespoons tomato paste

- 1 garlic clove (finely minced) - may cause wind and odour for ostomates

- 1/2 brown onion (finely minced) - may cause wind and odour for ostomates

- 1 1/2 teaspoons paprika (or sumach)

- 1 teaspoon cumin

- 1/4 teaspoon stevia powder

- salt and pepper to taste

- olive oil spray

- 6 free range eggs

- 1 tablespoon freshly chopped parsley

Instructions

Heat the cast iron pot on a medium heat.

Spray with olive oil.

Add fresh onion and garlic cook until soft.

Add tomatoes, red pepper and tomato paste blend well.

Add spices and stevia and mix into the sauce.

Salt and pepper to taste.

Turn heat down to low heat.

Crack eggs on top of the sauce leaving space between them.

Place a lid on the pot and simmer the pan for 10-15 minutes until the eggs are the way you like them (best served slightly soft).

Scoop sauce and eggs into ceramic dishes with the egg on top of the sauce, and serve immediately with a sprinkle of fresh parsley and soft white Turkish bread.

NOTE: for best results cook in cast iron cookware. NOTE: 3g Fiber content per serve includes white Turkish bread.

Creamy coconut apple porridge (Low Fiber)

Ingredients

- 1 large red apple (cored, peeled and chopped)

- 60 grams rice porridge

- 400 ml milk of your choice

- 1 teaspoon vanilla

- 1 tablespoon flaked coconut

- Topping:

- 2 teaspoons crushed cashew nuts (leave out for ostomates)

- 2 tablespoons coconut yoghurt

Instructions

Finely grate the apple and place all the **Ingredients** into a medium pan and simmer stirring regularly for 5-10 minutes until the mix is thick and creamy.

Leave to cool for a few minutes and top each serving with a tablespoon of coconut yoghurt and 1 teaspoon of crushed cashew nuts.

Curried carrot soup (Low Fiber)

Ingredients

- 1 tablespoon olive oil

- 1 teaspoon mustard seed

- 1/2 yellow onion, chopped (about 1/2 cup)

- 1 pound carrots, peeled and cut into 1/2-inch pieces

- 1 tablespoon plus 1 teaspoon peeled and chopped fresh ginger

- 1/2 jalapeno, seeded

- 2 teaspoons curry powder

- 5 cups low-sodium chicken stock, vegetable stock or broth

- 1/4 cup chopped fresh cilantro (fresh coriander), plus leaves for garnish

- 2 tablespoons fresh lime juice

- 1/2 teaspoon salt (optional)

- 3 tablespoons low-fat sour cream or fat-free plain yogurt

- Grated zest of 1 lime

Instructions

In a large saucepan, heat the olive oil over medium heat. Add the mustard seed. When the seeds just start to pop, after about 1 minute, add the onion and saute until soft and translucent, about 4 minutes. Add the carrots, ginger, jalapeno and curry powder and saute until the seasonings are fragrant, about 3 minutes. Add 3 cups of the stock, raise the heat to high and bring to a boil. Reduce the heat to medium-low and simmer, uncovered, until the carrots are tender, about 6 minutes.

In a blender or food processor, puree the soup in small batches until smooth and return to the saucepan. Note: The soup will be hot. Fill blender or processor no more than one-third full to avoid burns.

Stir in the remaining 2 cups stock. Return the soup to medium heat and reheat gently. Just before serving, stir in the chopped cilantro and lime juice. Season with the salt, if desired. Ladle into warmed individual bowls. Garnish with a drizzle of yogurt, a sprinkle of lime zest and cilantro leaves.

Potato soup with apples and Brie (Low fiber)

Ingredients

- 1 cup chopped yellow onion

- 1/4 cup sliced leek (white part only)

- 4 large Granny Smith apples, cored, peeled and quartered

- 2 cups low-sodium chicken broth

- 1 bay leaf

- 1/4 teaspoon dried thyme

- 3 cups fat-free evaporated milk

- 6 small potatoes, peeled and sliced (about 1/2 pound)

- 4 ounces Brie, cut into small cubes

- 1 large Granny Smith apple, cored and sliced thinly, for garnish

Instructions

Spray a soup pot with cooking spray. Add the onion, leeks and quartered apples. Saute over medium heat until softened, 5 to 7 minutes. Add the chicken broth, bay leaf and thyme. Bring to a boil, reduce heat to low and simmer for about 15 minutes. Remove the bay leaf. Turn off heat and set the mixture aside.

While the broth mixture is cooking, combine the evaporated milk and potatoes in a separate saucepan. Cook over medium heat until the potatoes are tender, 15 to 20 minutes. Stir frequently. Pour the potato mixture into the soup pot. Stir to mix evenly.

In a blender or food processor, puree the soup in small batches until smooth, adding the pieces of Brie while pureeing. Note: The soup will be hot. Fill blender or processor no more than one-third full to avoid burns.

Return pureed soup to pot and heat until warmed through. Ladle into individual bowls and garnish with thin slices of apple. Serve immediately.

Peanut Butter & Chia Berry Jam English Muffin

Ingredients

- ½ cup unsweetened mixed frozen berries
- 2 teaspoons chia seeds
- 2 teaspoons natural peanut butter
- 1 whole-wheat English muffin, toasted

Instructions

1. Microwave berries in a medium microwave-safe bowl for 30 seconds; stir and microwave 30 seconds more. Stir in chia seeds.
2. Spread peanut butter on the English muffin. Top with the berry-chia mixture.

Raspberry-Peach-Mango Smoothie Bowl

Ingredients

- 1 cup frozen mango chunks
- ¾ cup nonfat plain Greek yogurt
- ¼ cup reduced-fat milk
- 1 teaspoon vanilla extract
- ¼ ripe peach, sliced
- ⅓ cup raspberries
- 1 tablespoon sliced almonds, toasted if desired

- 1 tablespoon unsweetened coconut flakes, toasted if desired

- 1 teaspoon chia seeds

Instructions

1. Combine mango, yogurt, milk and vanilla in a blender. Puree until smooth.

2. Pour the smoothie into a bowl and top with peach slices, raspberries, almonds, coconut and chia seeds to taste.

Strawberry-Chocolate Smoothie

Ingredients

- 1 ½ cups frozen strawberries

- 1 cup chilled unsweetened chocolate almond milk, plus more if needed

- 1 tablespoon almond butter

- 1 tablespoon unsweetened cocoa powder

- 1 tablespoon honey

Instructions

1. Combine strawberries, almond milk, almond butter, cocoa and honey in a blender. Process until smooth, adding more almond milk, if needed, for desired consistency. Serve immediately.

Spinach-Avocado Smoothie

Ingredients

- 1 cup nonfat plain yogurt
- 1 cup fresh spinach
- 1 frozen banana
- ¼ avocado
- 2 tablespoons water
- 1 teaspoon honey

Instructions

1. Combine yogurt, spinach, banana, avocado, water and honey in a blender. Puree until smooth.

Peanut Butter-Banana English Muffin

Ingredients

- 1 whole-wheat English muffin, toasted
- 1 tablespoon peanut butter
- ½ banana, sliced
- Pinch of ground cinnamon

Instructions

1. Top English muffin with peanut butter, banana and cinnamon.

Blueberry Almond Chia Pudding

Ingredients

- ½ cup unsweetened almond milk or other nondairy milk beverage
- 2 tablespoons chia seeds
- 2 teaspoons pure maple syrup
- ⅛ teaspoon almond extract
- ½ cup fresh blueberries, divided
- 1 tablespoon toasted slivered almonds, divided

Instructions

1. Stir together almond milk (or other nondairy milk beverage), chia, maple syrup

and almond extract in a small bowl. Cover and refrigerate for at least 8 hours and up to 3 days.

2. When ready to serve, stir the pudding well. Spoon about half the pudding into a serving glass (or bowl) and top with half the blueberries and almonds. Add the rest of the pudding and top with the remaining blueberries and almonds.

Tips

To make ahead: Refrigerate pudding (Step 1) for up to 3 days. Finish with Step 2 just before serving.

Raspberry Yogurt Cereal Bowl

Ingredients

- 1 cup nonfat plain yogurt
- ½ cup mini shredded-wheat cereal
- ¼ cup fresh raspberries
- 2 teaspoons mini chocolate chips
- 1 teaspoon pumpkin seeds
- ¼ teaspoon ground cinnamon

Instructions

1. Place yogurt in a bowl and top with shredded wheat, raspberries, chocolate chips, pumpkin seeds and cinnamon.

DELICIOUS LUNCH RECIPES SUGGESTION FOR YOU

Low Fiber Lunch Recipe Suggestions

Baked cod with lemon and capers

Ingredients

- 4 cod fillets, each 6 ounces

- 1 lemon

- 1 teaspoon low-sodium chicken-flavored bouillon granules

- 1 cup hot tap water

- 1 tablespoon butter, softened

- 1 tablespoon all-purpose flour

- 4 teaspoons capers, rinsed and drained

Instructions

Heat the oven to 350 F. Spray 4 squares of foil with cooking spray.

Place 1 cod fillet on each foil square. Cut lemon in half. Squeeze the juice from one half over the fish. Cut the other half into slices, place over the fish and seal the foil.

Bake in the oven until the fish is opaque throughout when tested with the tip of a knife, about 20 minutes.

In a small bowl, add the chicken bouillon granules and the hot tap water. Stir until the granules dissolve. Set aside.

In another small bowl, mix the butter and flour together. Transfer to a heavy saucepan. Stir over moderate heat until the butter-flour mixture melts. Add the bouillon to the butter mixture and continue to stir until thickened. Add the capers and remove from the heat. Pour over the fish and serve.

Balsamic feta chicken

Ingredients

- 6 chicken breasts, 4 ounces each
- 1/2 cup balsamic vinegar
- 2 tablespoons brown sugar
- 1 tablespoon olive oil

- 1 tablespoon paprika

- 1 teaspoon chopped fresh thyme

- 1/2 teaspoon kosher salt

- 1/4 teaspoon dry mustard

- 6 tablespoons crumbled feta cheese

Instructions

Heat the oven to 375 F. Lightly coat a baking sheet or baking dish with cooking spray or olive oil.

In a medium bowl, combine the chicken breasts, vinegar, brown sugar, oil, paprika, thyme, salt and mustard. Using tongs, coat the chicken. Marinate the chicken breasts for at least 20 minutes in the refrigerator.

Place the marinaded chicken breasts on the baking sheet and bake for 15 minutes or until chicken reaches an internal temperature of 165 F. Sprinkle each chicken breast with 1 tablespoon cheese and serve.

White sea bass with dill relish

Ingredients

- 1 1/2 tablespoons chopped white onion
- 1 teaspoon pickled baby capers, drained
- 1 1/2 teaspoons chopped fresh dill
- 1 teaspoon Dijon mustard
- 1 teaspoon lemon juice

- 4 white sea bass fillets, each 4 ounces

- 1 lemon, cut in quarters

Instructions

Heat the oven to 375 F. In a small bowl, add the onion, capers, dill, mustard and lemon juice. Stir to mix well.

Place each fillet on a square of aluminum foil. Squeeze 1 lemon wedge over each fillet and spread 1/4 of the dill relish over each piece.

Wrap the aluminum foil around the fish and bake until the fish is opaque throughout when tested with a tip of a knife, 10 to 12 minutes. Serve immediately.

Thai peanut beef

Ingredients

- 5 tablespoons soy sauce
- 2 tablespoons creamy peanut butter
- 2 tablespoons brown sugar
- 2 tablespoons chopped scallions
- 2 tablespoons chopped cilantro
- 1 tablespoon vinegar
- 1 tablespoon ginger powder
- 1/2 teaspoon red pepper flakes
- 1/4 teaspoon salt

- 8 ounces beef tenderloin, cleaned and cut into 1-ounce pieces

- 1 tablespoon sesame oil

Instructions

In a small bowl, combine the soy sauce, peanut butter, sugar, scallions, cilantro, vinegar, ginger powder, red pepper flakes and salt. Mix well. Place beef tenderloins into marinade mixture and refrigerate for at least 30 minutes.

Heat a medium saute pan over medium-high heat. Once pan is hot, add oil and beef tenderloin. Sear beef on both sides. Cook thoroughly to an internal temperature of 145 F. Add the reserved marinade to the pan, reduce heat and cook until marinade is slightly thickened.

Swordfish with roasted lemons

Ingredients

- 2 lemons, quartered, seeds removed
- 1 tablespoon sugar
- 1/4 teaspoon sea salt
- 4 swordfish fillets, each 6 ounces
- 1/2 teaspoon canola oil
- 1/2 teaspoon chopped garlic
- 1/4 cup chopped parsley

Instructions

Heat the oven to 375 F.

In a small bowl, add the lemon wedges, sugar and salt. Toss gently to coat evenly. Place the lemons in a shallow baking dish and cover with aluminum foil. Roast until soft and slightly browned, about 1 hour.

Heat the broiler (grill). Position the rack 4 inches from the heat source. Lightly coat a baking pan with cooking spray.

Place the fish fillets in the prepared baking pan. Brush with canola oil and top with garlic. Broil (grill) until the fish is opaque throughout when tested with the tip of a knife, about 5 minutes on each side.

Transfer the fish to individual plates. Squeeze 1 roasted lemon wedge over each fillet and sprinkle with parsley. Serve with another roasted lemon wedge on the side.

Sweet potato souffle

Ingredients

- 1/2 cup panko breadcrumbs
- 4 cups mashed sweet potatoes
- 1/2 teaspoon unsalted butter
- 1 teaspoon chopped fresh thyme
- 1/4 teaspoon salt and ground black pepper, mixed
- Pinch of ground nutmeg
- 1 1/3 cup skim milk
- 1 1/2 tablespoon cornstarch

- 1/2 cup grated Gruyere cheese

- 3 egg whites

Instructions

Heat the oven to 375 F. Lightly coat 6 (8-ounce) ramekins with cooking spray and sprinkle with panko breadcrumbs. Place the ramekins on a baking sheet.

Heat a medium saute pan over medium heat. Add the sweet potatoes, butter, thyme, salt and pepper, and nutmeg.

In a small bowl, combine milk and cornstarch to form a slurry. Add the slurry to the pan and bring to a light boil while whisking frequently. Reduce heat and stir in the cheese. Once the cheese is melted, remove from heat and let the mixture cool.

In a medium bowl, whip the egg whites with an electric mixer until firm peaks form. Carefully fold the sweet potato mixture into the egg whites. Place equal amounts of the mixture into the ramekins and bake for approximately 20 minutes or until the center is firm and slightly golden brown.

Barbecued pork tenderloin

Ingredients

- 2 teaspoons firmly packed brown sugar
- 1 teaspoon ground allspice
- 1 teaspoon ground cinnamon
- 1/2 teaspoon ground ginger

- 1/2 teaspoon onion powder

- 1/2 teaspoon garlic powder

- 1/4 teaspoon cayenne pepper

- 1/8 teaspoon ground cloves

- 3/4 teaspoon salt, divided

- 1/2 teaspoon freshly ground black pepper

- 1 pork tenderloin, about 1 pound, trimmed of visible fat

- 2 teaspoons white vinegar

- 1 1/2 teaspoons dark honey

- 1 teaspoon tomato paste

Instructions

In a small bowl, combine the brown sugar, allspice, cinnamon, ginger, onion powder, garlic powder, cayenne pepper, cloves, 1/2 teaspoon of the salt and the black pepper. Rub the spice mixture over the pork and let stand for 15 minutes.

In another small bowl, combine the vinegar, honey, tomato paste and the remaining 1/4 teaspoon salt. Whisk to blend. Set aside.

Prepare a hot fire in a charcoal grill or heat a gas grill or broiler (grill) to medium-high or 400 F. Away from the heat source, lightly coat the grill rack or broiler pan with cooking spray. Position the cooking rack 4 to 6 inches from the heat source.

Place the pork on the grill rack or broiler pan. Grill or broil at medium-high heat, turning several times, until browned on all sides, 3 to 4 minutes total. Remove to a cooler part of the grill or reduce the heat and continue cooking for 14 to 16 minutes.

Baste with the vinegar-honey glaze and continue cooking until the pork is slightly pink inside and an instant-read thermometer inserted into the thickest part reads 160 F, 3 to 4 minutes longer. Transfer to a cutting board and let cool for 5 minutes before slicing.

To serve, slice the pork tenderloin crosswise into 16 pieces and arrange on a warmed serving platter, or divide the slices among individual plates.

High Fiber Lunch Recipe Suggestions

Avocado Toast with Burrata

Ingredients

- 1 slice whole-grain toast (3/4 inch thick)
- ½ large ripe avocado, thinly sliced
- 1 teaspoon lemon juice
- ⅛ teaspoon kosher salt
- ⅛ teaspoon ground pepper
- 1 ½ ounces burrata or fresh mozzarella cheese
- 1 teaspoon finely sliced fresh basil

- 1 teaspoon minced fresh chives
- Pinch of Aleppo pepper

Instructions

1. Top toast with avocado. Drizzle with lemon juice and sprinkle with salt and pepper. Top with burrata (or mozzarella), basil, chives and Aleppo pepper.

Chicken, Avocado & Quinoa Bowls with Herb Dressing

Ingredients

Roasted Chicken Thighs

- 5 boneless, skinless chicken thighs (about 1 1/4 pounds), trimmed
- ½ teaspoon ground pepper
- ¼ teaspoon salt

Quinoa

- 3 cups low-sodium chicken broth
- 1 tablespoon extra-virgin olive oil
- ¼ teaspoon salt
- 1 ½ cups quinoa

Italian Dressing

- ¾ cup red-wine vinegar
- 5 tablespoons water

- 1 ½ tablespoons sugar

- 1 tablespoon Dijon mustard

- 1 large clove garlic

- 2 teaspoons dried basil

- 2 teaspoons dried oregano

- ½ teaspoon salt

- ½ teaspoon ground pepper

- 1 ¾ cups extra-virgin olive oil

Toppings

- 1 (15 ounce) can chickpeas, rinsed

- 1 avocado, sliced

- 6 radishes, thinly sliced

- 1 cup sprouts or shoots

- ¼ cup toasted seeds or chopped nuts

Instructions

1. To prepare chicken: Preheat oven to 425 degrees F. Place chicken on a baking sheet. Sprinkle with 1/2 teaspoon ground pepper and 1/4 teaspoon salt. Roast the chicken until an instant-read thermometer inserted in the thickest part registers 165 degrees F, 14 to 16 minutes. Slice 4 thighs. (Reserve 1 thigh for another use.)

2. Meanwhile, prepare quinoa: Combine broth, 1 tablespoon oil and 1/4 teaspoon salt in a large saucepan. Bring to a simmer over high heat. Stir in quinoa and return to a simmer. Reduce heat and simmer until the

quinoa has absorbed all the liquid and the grains have burst, 15 to 20 minutes. Remove from heat, cover and let stand for 5 minutes. (Reserve 2 cups for another use.)

3. To prepare dressing: Combine vinegar, water, sugar, mustard, garlic, basil, oregano, salt and pepper in a blender. Puree until smooth. With the motor running, slowly add oil and puree until creamy. (Transfer 1 3/4 cups to a large mason jar and refrigerate for up to 1 week.)

4. To assemble bowls: Divide 3 cups quinoa among 4 large shallow bowls. Top with the chicken, chickpeas, avocado, radishes and sprouts (or shoots); sprinkle with seeds (or nuts). Drizzle with 3/4 cup dressing.

Tips

To make ahead: Prepare chicken (Step 1) and quinoa (Step 2); refrigerate separately for up to 5 days. Prepare dressing (Step 3); refrigerate for up to 1 week.

Meal-Prep Roasted Vegetable Bowls with Pesto

Ingredients

- 3 tablespoons extra-virgin olive oil, divided
- ½ teaspoon garlic powder
- ¼ teaspoon salt
- ¼ teaspoon ground pepper
- 4 cups broccoli florets

- 2 medium red bell peppers, quartered

- 1 cup sliced red onion

- 3 cups cooked brown rice

- 1 (15 ounce) can chickpeas, rinsed

- 4 tablespoons prepared pesto

Instructions

1. Preheat oven to 450 degrees F.

2. Whisk 2 tablespoons oil, garlic powder, salt and pepper together in a large bowl. Add broccoli, peppers and onion; toss to coat. Transfer to a large rimmed baking sheet and roast, stirring once, until the vegetables are tender, about 20 minutes. Chop the peppers when cool enough to handle.

3. Stir the remaining 1 tablespoon oil into rice. Place about 3/4 cup of the rice in each of four 2-cup microwave-safe, lidded containers. Divide chickpeas and the roasted vegetables among the bowls. Top each with 1 tablespoon pesto.

4. To reheat: Microwave each container on High until heated through, 1 to 2 minutes.

Halloumi Grain Bowls With Figs and Charred Lemon Dressing

Ingredients

- 1 cup uncooked pearled farro

- 1/4 cup plus 2 tsp olive oil, divided

- 2 large lemons, halved crosswise

- 2 1/2 tsp honey or hot honey

- 1 tsp kosher salt

- 1 medium bunch curly kale, stemmed and torn (about 8 cups)

- 1 cup dried figs, quartered, or halved if small

- 1 8.8-oz. block Halloumi cheese, cut crosswise into 12 (1/4-in.-thick) slices

- 1/4 cup sliced almonds, toasted

- 1/4 cup torn fresh mint

Instructions

1. Bring a medium saucepan filled with water to a boil. Add farro; reduce heat to medium

to maintain a gentle boil. Cook, stirring occasionally, until tender, 15 to 20 minutes. Drain.

2. Meanwhile, heat 2 teaspoons oil in a large nonstick skillet over medium. Add lemon halves, cut side down. Cook, undisturbed, until cut sides are charred, about 3 minutes. Remove from heat. Let lemon halves cool slightly, about 5 minutes. Wipe skillet clean.

3. Squeeze lemon halves into a medium bowl to measure 1/4 cup juice. Whisk in honey and 1/2 teaspoon salt. Gradually drizzle in remaining 1/4 cup oil, whisking constantly until combined.

4. Place kale, 1 tablespoon lemon dressing, and remaining 1/2 teaspoon salt in a large bowl. Using your hands, massage kale until

softened and wilted, about 2 minutes. Add drained farro and figs to bowl. Drizzle with about 1/3 cup lemon dressing; toss to coat.

5. Heat cleaned nonstick skillet over medium-high. Pat cheese slices dry. Add cheese to skillet in a single layer; cook until golden brown on both sides, 2 to 3 minutes per side.

6. Serve farro and kale mixture in bowls topped with cheese, almonds, and mint. Drizzle with remaining dressing. Serve warm or at room temperature.

Superfood Lentil Salad

Ingredients

- 2 large zucchini, cut into 1-inch chunks (3 cups)

- ⅓ cup plus 2 tablespoons olive oil, divided

- 1 ½ teaspoons kosher salt, divided

- ½ teaspoon freshly ground black pepper, divided

- ⅓ cup golden raisins

- ¼ teaspoons crushed red pepper

- ¼ cup apple cider vinegar, divided

- 1 cup dried beluga lentils or French green lentils, rinsed

- 1 clove garlic, smashed

- 2 scallions, trimmed and thinly sliced, white and green parts separated

- ½ cup unsalted roasted sunflower seeds, plus more for serving

- ½ teaspoon Dijon mustard

- Microgreens or sprouts, for serving

Instructions

1. Preheat broiler with rack in upper third. Stir zucchini, 2 tablespoons oil, ½ teaspoon salt, and ¼ teaspoon black pepper on a rimmed baking sheet; spread in an even layer. Broil until charred in spots and softened, 8 to 10 minutes. Transfer to a large bowl. Add raisins, crushed red pepper, and 2 tablespoons vinegar; stir to combine. Set aside.

2. Bring 2 cups water, lentils, garlic, and ½ teaspoon salt to a boil in a saucepan over

medium-high. Cover and reduce heat to low. Cook until lentils are just tender, about 20 minutes. Drain well; discard garlic. Let cool for 10 minutes. Transfer to bowl with zucchini.

3. Place white and light green scallion slices, sunflower seeds, mustard, and remaining 2 tablespoons vinegar, ½ teaspoon salt, and ¼ teaspoon black pepper in a food processor. Pulse until a coarse paste forms. Scrape sides of bowl and add remaining ⅓ cup oil. Pulse until incorporated, 2 to 3 pulses.

4. Stir vinaigrette into lentil mixture with sliced dark green scallion tops. Top with microgreens and sunflower seeds.

Turkey-Pumpkin Chili

Ingredients

- 2 tablespoons olive oil

- 1 small yellow onion, chopped

- 1 pound 93% lean ground turkey

- 1 tablespoon plus 1 tsp. ground coriander

- 2 ½ teaspoons smoked paprika

- 1 ½ teaspoons kosher salt

- 2 15-oz. cans cannellini beans, drained and rinsed

- 1 15-oz. can pumpkin puree

- 1 ½ cups low-sodium chicken broth

- Hot sauce, sour cream, and sliced scallions, for serving

Instructions

1. Heat oil in a medium heavy-bottomed pot over medium-high. Add onion and cook, stirring occasionally, until tender, about 5 minutes. Stir in turkey, coriander, paprika, and salt; cook, stirring occasionally, until turkey is browned, about 5 minutes.

2. Stir beans, pumpkin, 1¾ cups water, and broth into turkey mixture. Bring to a simmer over medium-high, stirring occasionally. Reduce heat to medium and cook, stirring often, until heated through, about 15 minutes. Top with hot sauce, sour cream, and scallions.

Sweet Potato and Kale Tortilla Soup

Ingredients

- 3 tablespoons olive oil, divided
- 1 small yellow onion, chopped (about 1 cup)
- ¾ teaspoon fine sea salt
- 1 tablespoon chili powder
- 1 tablespoon ground cumin
- 2 teaspoons ground coriander
- 2 large garlic cloves, chopped (about 1½ Tbsp.)

- 1 (28-oz.) can whole peeled tomatoes, undrained

- 1 large sweet potato (about 1 lb., 6 oz.), peeled and cut into 1-inch pieces (about 4½ cups)

- 4 cups vegetable broth

- 2 cups water

- 6 (6-inch) corn tortillas

- 1 small bunch kale (about 5 oz.), ribs removed and leaves torn into bite-size pieces (about 2 packed cups)

- 2 cooked and shredded chicken (from 1 [3-lb.] rotisserie chicken) (optional)

- Freshly ground black pepper

- Lime wedges, for serving

Instructions

1. Preheat oven to 400 F with an oven rack in upper position.

2. Heat 2 tablespoons of the oil in a large pot over medium-high. Add onion, and season with ¼ teaspoon of the salt; cook, stirring occasionally, until softened, about 3 minutes. Add chili powder, cumin, coriander, and garlic, and cook, stirring often, until fragrant, about 1 minute. Add tomatoes with juices, and cook, stirring often and breaking up with a spoon, until slightly reduced, 2 to 4 minutes.

3. Add sweet potato, broth, and water, and bring to a boil. Reduce heat to medium-low,

and simmer, partially covered, until potatoes are fork tender, 12 to 15 minutes.

4. Meanwhile, brush remaining 1 tablespoon oil on both sides of tortillas; season with ¼ teaspoon of the salt. Stack tortillas, and cut into ½-inch strips; place in a single layer on a rimmed baking sheet. Bake in preheated oven on top rack until golden brown, 12 to 15 minutes, tossing halfway through.

5. Stir kale into soup, and cook, covered, until wilted, 3 to 5 minutes. Stir 2 handfuls of tortilla strips into soup, and, if desired, chicken; cook until soup is heated through, about 2 minutes. Season with remaining ¼ teaspoon salt and several grinds black pepper. Serve with lime wedges, and top with remaining tortilla strips.

Creamy Miso White Bean Soup

Ingredients

- ¼ cup extra-virgin olive oil, divided

- 1 cup chopped yellow onion

- 3 15-ounce cans cannellini beans, drained and rinsed

- 4 cups vegetable broth

- 1 teaspoon kosher salt

- 1 tablespoon rosemary leaves, divided

- 3 tablespoons white miso

- 2 tablespoons unsalted butter

- 1 tablespoon sherry vinegar

Instructions

1. Heat 2 tablespoons of the olive oil in a large pot over medium-high. Add onion, and cook, stirring occasionally, until translucent, about 5 minutes. Stir in cannellini beans, vegetable broth, salt, and 2 teaspoons of the rosemary leaves, and bring to a boil over medium-high. Reduce heat to medium, and simmer until beans are very soft, about 15 minutes.

2. Transfer bean mixture to a blender; add miso. Secure lid on blender; remove center piece to allow steam to escape, and place a clean towel over opening. Process until smooth, about 30 seconds. Transfer mixture back to pot over medium-low. Add butter

and vinegar, and stir until butter melts. Serve immediately topped with remaining 2 tablespoons olive oil and 1 teaspoon rosemary leaves.

DINNER RECIPES SUGGESTION FOR YOU

Low Fiber Recipe Suggestions

Blackened sole

Ingredients

- 2 teaspoons paprika

- 2 teaspoons onion powder

- 2 teaspoons salt

- 1 teaspoon thyme

- 1 tablespoon garlic powder

- 1 tablespoon sugar

- 1 teaspoon pepper

- 1 teaspoon oregano

- 1/2 teaspoon cumin

- 1/2 teaspoon cayenne pepper

- 1 teaspoon olive oil

- 2 sole fillets, 4 ounces each

Instructions

In a small bowl or small zip-close bag, combine the herbs and spices. Season one side of each sole fillet with 1 teaspoon of seasoning mixture on the top side of the fillet — not the skin side.

Heat a large saute pan on medium-high heat; add olive oil. Cook fillets on the seasoned side first for about 1 minute. Flip the fillets and lower the heat to medium. Cover for about 2 to 3 minutes. Fillets should flake when done. Use a meat thermometer to make sure the internal temperature of the fillet has reached 145 F before serving.

Broiled grouper with teriyaki sauce

Ingredients

- 1 tablespoon reduced-sodium teriyaki sauce

- 1/2 teaspoon minced garlic

- 2 grouper fillets, each 4 ounces

- 2 lemon wedges

- 1/4 teaspoon Italian seasoning

Instructions

In a small bowl, whisk together the teriyaki sauce and garlic.

Lightly spray a baking pan with cooking spray. Place the grouper fillets in the pan. Brush the teriyaki marinade on both sides of the fillets. Cover and refrigerate for at least 15 minutes to marinate the fish.

Heat the broiler or grill. Position the rack 4 inches from the heat source.

Broil or grill until the fish is not transparent, also called opaque, throughout when tested with a tip of a knife, about 5 to 10 minutes. Remove from the broiler or grill.

Squeeze 1 lemon wedge over each fillet. Then sprinkle with Italian seasoning.

Serve right away.

Chicken Parmesan

Ingredients

- 4 chicken breasts (4 ounces each)
- 2 egg whites
- 1 cup panko breadcrumbs
- 1/2 cup grated Parmesan cheese
- 2 teaspoons dry basil
- 2 teaspoons dry oregano
- 1 teaspoon garlic powder
- 1 teaspoon onion powder

- 2 cups reduced-sodium marinara sauce

- 1/2 cup shredded part-skim mozzarella cheese

Instructions

Heat the oven to 375 F. Coat a baking sheet with cooking spray.

Pound out each chicken breast to 1/4-inch thickness. Set aside. Place the egg whites in a medium bowl. In another medium bowl, combine the breadcrumbs, Parmesan, basil, oregano, garlic powder and onion powder. Dip each chicken breast into the egg whites, then dredge in the breadcrumb mixture. Lay fillets on the baking sheet.

Bake for 15 to 20 minutes or until chicken is golden brown and internal temperature is 165 F. Top chicken with marinara and mozzarella cheese. Serve.

Fish Veracruz

Ingredients

- 2 pounds whitefish fillets, such as tilapia, cod, sole, pollock or halibut

- 1/4 cup lime juice

- 1/2 tablespoon canola oil

- 1 small onion, peeled and sliced

- 1 small green bell pepper, seeded and cut into strips

- 1/4 cup jalapeno pepper, seeded and sliced

- 2 cups fresh salsa or pico de gallo

- 1/2 cup no-salt-added tomato sauce

- 1/2 cup sliced ripe olives

- 1 tablespoon capers

- 4 tablespoons chopped fresh cilantro or 4 teaspoons dried cilantro

- 1 lime cut into 8 wedges

Instructions

In a 9-by-13-inch baking pan, arrange fish. Sprinkle with lime juice. Cover and refrigerate for at least 20 minutes.

Preheat oven to 425 F. In a large, nonstick skillet, heat oil over medium-high heat. Add onion, bell pepper and jalapeno pepper. Cook and stir a bit for 2 minutes, or until vegetables are tender yet crisp.

Stir in salsa, tomato sauce, olives and capers. Bring to a boil. Reduce heat and simmer for 1 minute.

Pour the sauce over the fish and bake for about 20 minutes, or until fish flakes easily with a fork.

Remove fish and vegetables from the pan with a slotted spatula. Serve with cilantro and lime wedges.

Grilled salmon

Ingredients

- 2 fillets (4 ounces each) salmon

- 1/2 teaspoon salt

- 1/2 teaspoon black pepper

Instructions

Heat a grill or cast-iron skillet to medium heat. Spray cooking spray on the cooking surface and on one side of the salmon fillets. Season the sprayed side of the fillets with salt and pepper. Lay the fillets, seasoned-side down, on the cooking surface and cook for about 3 minutes. Turn the fillets 90 degrees and cook for another 3 minutes.

Spray the top of the fillets with cooking spray and flip them over. Cook for about 3 minutes, turn 90 degrees, and cook for another 3 minutes until the fish is cooked through.

Pork tenderloin with apples and blue cheese

Ingredients

- 1 pound pork tenderloin

- 1/2 teaspoon white pepper

- 2 teaspoons black pepper

- 1/4 teaspoon cayenne pepper

- 1 teaspoon paprika

- 2 teaspoons canola oil

- 2 apples, sliced

- 1/2 cup white wine or 1/2 cup unsweetened apple juice

- 1/4 cup (about 1 ounce) crumbled blue cheese

Instructions

Heat oven to 350 F. Trim tenderloin of all fat and silvery membrane. Season with spices.

In a large skillet over medium-high heat, add oil and put tenderloin in the pan. Sear each side, using tongs to turn the meat. Transfer meat to a roasting pan and cook in oven for 15 to 20 minutes, until internal temperature reaches 155 F. Remove from oven and transfer tenderloin to a platter. Cover with foil and let rest.

Add apples to roasting pan and saute on stovetop until dark brown. Add wine (or juice) and simmer until liquid is reduced by half.

Slice pork, spoon apples over top and sprinkle with blue cheese. Serve.

Roasted salmon with maple glaze

Ingredients

- 1/4 cup maple syrup

- 1 garlic clove, minced

- 1/4 cup balsamic vinegar

- 2 pounds salmon, cut into 6 equal-sized fillets

- 1/4 teaspoon kosher or sea salt

- 1/8 teaspoon fresh cracked black pepper

- Fresh mint or parsley for garnish

Instructions

Heat the oven to 450 F. Lightly coat a baking pan with cooking spray.

In a small saucepan over low heat, mix together the maple syrup, garlic and balsamic vinegar. Heat just until hot and remove from heat. Pour half of the mixture into a small bowl to use for basting, and reserve the rest for later.

Pat the salmon dry. Place skin-side down on the baking sheet. Baste the salmon with the maple syrup mixture. Bake about 10 minutes, baste again with maple syrup mixture and bake for another 5 minutes. Continue to baste and bake until fish flakes easily, about 20 to 25 minutes total.

Transfer the salmon fillets to plates. Sprinkle with salt and black pepper, and top with reserved maple syrup mixture. Garnish with fresh mint or parsley and serve immediately.

High Fiber Recipe Suggestions

Easy Pea & Spinach Carbonara

Ingredients

- 1 ½ tablespoons extra-virgin olive oil
- ½ cup panko breadcrumbs, preferably whole-wheat
- 1 small clove garlic, minced
- 8 tablespoons grated Parmesan cheese, divided
- 3 tablespoons finely chopped fresh parsley
- 3 large egg yolks
- 1 large egg

- ½ teaspoon ground pepper

- ¼ teaspoon salt

- 1 (9 ounce) package fresh tagliatelle or linguine

- 8 cups baby spinach

- 1 cup peas (fresh or frozen)

Instructions

1. Put 10 cups of water in a large pot and bring to a boil over high heat.

2. Meanwhile, heat oil in a large skillet over medium-high heat. Add breadcrumbs and garlic; cook, stirring frequently, until toasted, about 2 minutes. Transfer to a small bowl and stir in 2 tablespoons Parmesan and parsley. Set aside.

3. Whisk the remaining 6 tablespoons Parmesan, egg yolks, egg, pepper and salt in a medium bowl.

4. Cook pasta in the boiling water, stirring occasionally, for 1 minute. Add spinach and peas and cook until the pasta is tender, about 1 minute more. Reserve 1/4 cup of the cooking water. Drain and place in a large bowl.

5. Slowly whisk the reserved cooking water into the egg mixture. Gradually add the mixture to the pasta, tossing with tongs to combine. Serve topped with the reserved breadcrumb mixture.

Quinoa Chickpea Salad with Roasted Red Pepper Hummus Dressing

Ingredients

- 2 tablespoons hummus, original or roasted red pepper flavor
- 1 tablespoon lemon juice
- 1 tablespoon chopped roasted red pepper
- 2 cups mixed salad greens
- ½ cup cooked quinoa
- ½ cup chickpeas, rinsed
- 1 tablespoon unsalted sunflower seeds
- 1 tablespoon chopped fresh parsley

- Pinch of salt

- Pinch of ground pepper

Instructions

1. Stir hummus, lemon juice and red peppers in a small dish. Thin with water to desired consistency for dressing.

2. Arrange greens, quinoa and chickpeas in a large bowl. Top with sunflower seeds, parsley, salt and pepper. Serve with the dressing.

Sautéed Broccoli with Peanut Sauce

Ingredients

- 8 cups broccoli florets (2-inch pieces)
- 2 tablespoons toasted sesame oil
- 1 cup sliced red bell pepper
- ½ cup sliced yellow onion
- 3 medium cloves garlic, chopped
- 3 tablespoons smooth natural peanut butter
- 2 ½ tablespoons reduced-sodium tamari
- 2 tablespoons rice vinegar
- 1 tablespoon light brown sugar
- 1 teaspoon cornstarch
- 1 tablespoon toasted sesame seeds

Instructions

1. Bring 1 inch of water to a boil in a large pot fitted with a steamer basket. Add broccoli, cover and cook until tender-crisp, 3 to 4 minutes.

2. Meanwhile, heat oil in a large skillet over medium-high heat. Add bell pepper, onion and garlic; cook, stirring often, until the vegetables begin to soften, about 3 minutes. Add the steamed broccoli and cook, stirring, for 3 minutes.

3. Whisk peanut butter, tamari, vinegar, sugar and cornstarch in a small bowl until smooth. Stir into the vegetables. Cook, stirring, until the sauce thickens, about 1 minute. Sprinkle with sesame seeds.

Loaded Gentle Black Bean Nacho Soup

Ingredients

- 1 (18-ounce) carton low-sodium pureed vegetable or lentil soup
- ⅛ teaspoon smoked paprika (optional, for flavor)
- ½ teaspoon lime juice
- ½ cup cooked and finely chopped zucchini or carrots
- 2 tablespoons shredded mild cheese (e.g., mozzarella or Monterey Jack)
- ½ medium avocado, diced
- 2 small soft tortilla strips, lightly toasted

Instructions

1. Pour soup into a small saucepan and stir in paprika, if using. Heat according to package directions. Stir in lime juice.
2. Divide the soup between 2 bowls and top with cooked zucchini or carrots, cheese, and avocado.
3. Serve with soft tortilla strips or enjoy as is.

Cheesy Spinach-&-Artichoke Stuffed Spaghetti Squash

Ingredients

- 1 (2 1/2 to 3 pound) spaghetti squash, cut in half lengthwise and seeds removed

- 3 tablespoons water, divided

- 1 (5 ounce) package baby spinach

- 1 (10 ounce) package frozen artichoke hearts, thawed and chopped

- 4 ounces reduced-fat cream cheese, cubed and softened

- ½ cup grated Parmesan cheese, divided

- ¼ teaspoon salt

- ¼ teaspoon ground pepper

- Crushed red pepper & chopped fresh basil for garnish

Instructions

1. Place squash cut-side down in a microwave-safe dish; add 2 tablespoons water.

Microwave, uncovered, on High until tender, 10 to 15 minutes. (Alternatively, place squash halves cut-side down on a rimmed baking sheet. Bake at 400 degrees F until tender, 40 to 50 minutes.)

2. Meanwhile, combine spinach and the remaining 1 tablespoon water in a large skillet over medium heat. Cook, stirring occasionally, until wilted, 3 to 5 minutes. Drain and transfer to a large bowl.

3. Position rack in upper third of oven; preheat broiler.

4. Use a fork to scrape the squash from the shells into the bowl. Place the shells on a baking sheet. Stir artichoke hearts, cream cheese, 1/4 cup Parmesan, salt and pepper into the squash mixture. Divide it between

the squash shells and top with the remaining 1/4 cup Parmesan. Broil until the cheese is golden brown, about 3 minutes. Sprinkle with crushed red pepper and basil, if desired.

Spaghetti & Chicken Meatballs with No-Cook Tomato Sauce

Ingredients

- 8 ounces whole-wheat spaghetti

- 4 cups chopped ripe tomatoes (about 1 3/4 pounds)

- 1 cup chopped fresh basil, plus more for garnish

- 3 cloves garlic, minced

- 3 tablespoons extra-virgin olive oil, divided

- 16 fully cooked refrigerated Italian-style chicken meatballs (see Tip)

- ¼ cup finely grated Parmesan cheese

Instructions

1. Bring a large pot of water to a boil. Cook spaghetti according to package directions. Drain.

2. Meanwhile, combine tomatoes, basil, garlic and 2 tablespoons oil in a medium bowl.

3. Heat the remaining 1 tablespoon oil in a large skillet over medium-high heat. Add meatballs and cook, stirring occasionally, until starting to brown, 3 to 5 minutes.

Remove from heat; add the tomato mixture and toss to coat. Serve the spaghetti with the meatballs and sauce, topped with Parmesan. Garnish with more basil, if desired.

Tips

Tip: Smart Shortcut: Keep a package of chicken meatballs on hand for a quick dinner hack. Look for them in your grocery store's meat department.

SNACK AND DESSERT RECIPE SUGGESTIONS

Raspberry-Jam Bites

Ingredients

- 16 ounces fresh raspberries (about 4 cups) *or* 3 1/2 cups frozen raspberries

- 2 tablespoons chia seeds

- 12 ounces dark chocolate (60-70%), chopped

Instructions

1. Line a large baking sheet with parchment paper. Place raspberries and chia seeds in a large bowl. Mash with a fork until the mixture is jammy. *(If using frozen raspberries,*

add 1/4 cup water, 1 tablespoon at a time, until the berries are loosened.) Scoop the mixture by heaping tablespoonfuls onto the prepared baking sheet. Freeze for at least 1 hour or up to 8 hours.

2. Line another baking sheet with parchment paper. Microwave chocolate in a medium microwave-safe bowl on Medium for 1 minute. Stir, then continue microwaving on Medium in 20-second intervals until melted, stopping to stir after each interval. *(Alternatively, place chocolate in the top of a double boiler over hot, but not boiling, water; stir until melted.)*

3. Remove the raspberry bites from the freezer. Using a fork, hold one bite over the melted chocolate and use a spoon to lightly coat it, allowing excess chocolate to drip back into

the bowl. Spoon about 1 teaspoon melted chocolate onto the parchment paper and place the coated bite on top. Repeat the process with the remaining bites. Use a spoon or fork to drizzle the tops of the bites with the remaining chocolate, if desired. Serve immediately or store in an airtight container in the freezer for up to 1 month.

Blueberry-Lemon Energy Balls

Ingredients

- ¾ cup walnuts

- ½ cup pitted dates

- ¼ cup dried blueberries

- ¾ cup old-fashioned rolled oats

- 2 tablespoons pure maple syrup

- 1 teaspoon grated lemon zest

- 1 tablespoon lemon juice

Instructions

1. Add walnuts, dates and blueberries to a food processor; process until chopped and combined, 7 to 10 seconds. Add oats, maple syrup and lemon juice. Continue processing until a smooth, thick paste forms, 20 to 30 seconds. Transfer the paste to a small bowl; add lemon zest and mix to combine. With your hands, form and roll the mixture into 18 small balls.

Banana Bran Muffins

Ingredients

- 1 large egg
- 1 large egg white
- ¾ cup packed light brown sugar
- 1 cup buttermilk
- 1 cup mashed banana, (2 medium bananas)
- 1 cup unprocessed wheat bran
- ¼ cup canola oil
- 1 teaspoon vanilla extract
- 1 ½ cups all-purpose flour
- 1 ½ teaspoons baking powder

- ½ teaspoon baking soda

- ½ teaspoon salt

- ½ teaspoon ground cinnamon

- 2 tablespoons chopped pecans, or walnuts

Instructions

1. Preheat oven to 400 degrees F. Coat 12 muffin cups with cooking spray.

2. Whisk egg, egg white and brown sugar in a medium bowl until smooth. Add buttermilk, banana, bran, oil and vanilla and whisk until blended. Whisk flour, baking powder, baking soda, salt and cinnamon in a large bowl. Make a well in the dry ingredients; add wet ingredients and stir with a rubber spatula until just combined.

3. Spoon batter into prepared muffin cups and sprinkle with nuts. Bake until tops spring back when touched lightly, 15 to 20 minutes. Loosen edges and turn muffins out onto a wire rack to cool.

Tips

DIY Muffin Cups: Make your next batch of muffins or cupcakes the ultimate grab-and-go treat by lining your tin with muffin liners. No liners? No problem. Use 5-inch squares of parchment paper, coat each muffin cup with cooking spray, and push each square into the cups using a small can or bottle, pressing the paper up the sides. (It's OK if some of the paper is sticking out over the rim.) Fill each cup as directed.

Kale Chips

Ingredients

- 1 large bunch kale, tough stems removed, leaves torn into pieces (about 16 cups)//
- 1 tablespoon extra-virgin olive oil
- ¼ teaspoon salt

Instructions

1. Position racks in upper third and center of oven; preheat to 400°F.

2. If kale is wet, very thoroughly pat dry with a clean kitchen towel; transfer to a large bowl. Drizzle the kale with oil and sprinkle with salt. Using your hands, massage the oil and salt onto the kale leaves to evenly coat.

Fill 2 large rimmed baking sheets with a layer of kale, making sure the leaves don't overlap. (If the kale won't all fit, make the chips in batches.)

3. Bake until most leaves are crisp, switching the pans back to front and top to bottom halfway through, 8 to 12 minutes total. (If baking a batch on just 1 sheet, start checking after 8 minutes to prevent burning.)

Chocolate-Peppermint Energy Balls

Ingredients

- 8 ounces dried pitted dates (about 1 3/4 cups)

- ⅔ cup rolled oats (see Tip)

- ½ cup creamy peanut butter

- 1 ½ ounces dark chocolate (70% cacao)

- ½ teaspoon salt

- 4 candy canes

Instructions

1. Process dates, oats, peanut butter, chocolate and salt in a food processor until well blended, about 45 seconds. Divide the mixture evenly into 16 balls, about 2 tablespoons each.

2. Break candy canes into large pieces; place in the food processor. Process until very finely chopped, about 1 minute. Transfer to a

medium bowl. Roll the balls in the crushed candy canes until well coated.

Tips

Tip: People with celiac disease or gluten sensitivity should use oats that are labeled "gluten-free," as oats are often cross-contaminated with wheat and barley.

To make ahead: Store in an airtight container at room temperature for up to 7 days.

Pineapple Spinach Smoothie

Ingredients

- ¼ cup pineapple juice

- ¼ cup water

- 2 cups baby spinach

- ½ cup frozen mango chunks

- ½ cup frozen pineapple chunks

Instructions

1. Combine pineapple juice and water in a blender, then add spinach, mango and pineapple. Puree until very smooth.

Peanut Butter and Banana Breakfast Sandwich

Ingredients

- 2 slices 100% whole wheat with honey bread

- 4 teaspoons reduced-fat creamy peanut butter

- 1 very small banana or 1/2 of a medium banana, sliced

Instructions

1. Toast bread. While toast is still warm, spread 2 teaspoons of the peanut butter on each slice. Arrange banana slices on one of the slices of peanut butter toast. Top with the other slice, peanut butter side down, to make a sandwich.

Blueberry-Pecan Energy Balls

Ingredients

- 1 ½ cups dried blueberries

- 1 ½ cups pecans

- 6 tablespoons cocoa nibs

- 6 tablespoons almond butter

- 3 tablespoons chia seeds

- 3 tablespoons pure maple syrup

- Pinch of salt

Instructions

1. Combine blueberries, pecans, cacao nibs, almond butter, chia seeds, maple syrup and

salt in a food processor. Pulse until finely chopped, 10 to 20 times, then process for about 1 minute, scraping down the sides as necessary, until the mixture is crumbly but can be pressed to form a cohesive ball.

2. With wet hands (to prevent the mixture from sticking to them), squeeze about 1 tablespoon of the mixture tightly between your hands and roll into a ball. Place in a storage container. Repeat with the remaining mixture.

Tips

To make ahead: Refrigerate for up to 1 week or freeze for up to 3 months.

Bagel Gone Bananas

Ingredients

- 2 tablespoons natural nut butter, such as almond, cashew or peanut
- 1 teaspoon honey
- Pinch of salt
- 1 whole-wheat bagel, split and toasted
- 1 small banana, sliced

Instructions

1. Stir together nut butter, honey and salt in a small bowl. Divide the mixture between bagel halves and top with banana slices.

Cranberry-Almond Energy Balls

Ingredients

- ¾ cup raw whole almonds

- ½ cup sweetened dried cranberries

- ¼ cup pitted dates

- ¾ cup old-fashioned rolled oats (see Tip)

- 2 tablespoons tahini

- 2 tablespoons fresh lemon juice

- 1 tablespoon pure maple syrup

Instructions

1. Add almonds, cranberries and dates to a large food processor; process on High until

the ingredients are broken into smaller pieces, 10 to 15 seconds. Add oats, tahini, lemon juice and maple syrup. Continue processing until a thick paste forms, 40 to 60 seconds. With your hands, roll the mixture into 25 balls, about 1 tablespoon per ball.

Pumpkin-Oatmeal Muffins

Ingredients

- 3 ½ cups old-fashioned rolled oats
- 1 ½ cups reduced-fat milk
- 1 cup unseasoned pumpkin puree
- ½ cup light brown sugar

- 1 ½ teaspoons vanilla extract

- 1 teaspoon baking powder

- 1 teaspoon pumpkin pie spice

- ¾ teaspoon salt

- 2 large eggs, lightly beaten

- ½ cup chopped pecans

Instructions

1. Preheat oven to 375 degrees F. Stir oats, milk, pumpkin, brown sugar, vanilla, baking powder, pumpkin pie spice, salt and eggs together in a large bowl until fully incorporated.

2. Lightly coat a 12-cup muffin tin with cooking spray. Spoon the batter into the

prepared muffin cups, filling each almost to the top. Sprinkle evenly with pecans.

3. Bake the muffins until a toothpick inserted in the center comes out clean, 25 to 30 minutes. Let cool in the pan for 10 minutes, then transfer to wire rack. Serve warm or at room temperature.

Tips

To make ahead: Wrap airtight and refrigerate for up to 2 days or freeze for up to 3 months.

Apple Pie Energy Balls

Ingredients

- ¾ cup Medjool dates, pitted and chopped

- ½ cup rolled oats

- ½ cup chopped dried apples

- ½ cup unsweetened almond butter

- ¼ cup chopped pecans, toasted

- 1 tablespoon ground cinnamon

Instructions

1. Soak ¾ cup dates in a small bowl of hot water until softened, 5 to 10 minutes. Drain.

2. Combine ½ cup oats, ½ cup dried apples, ½ cup almond butter, ¼ cup pecans, 1 tablespoon cinnamon and the soaked dates in a food processor; process until very finely chopped.

3. Roll the mixture into 12 balls (about 2 tablespoons each). Refrigerate for at least 15 minutes or up to 1 week.

Rosemary-Garlic Pecans

Ingredients

- 1 large egg white
- 3 tablespoons dried rosemary, finely chopped
- 2 teaspoons garlic salt
- 3 cups pecans

Instructions

1. Preheat oven to 250°F.

2. Whisk egg white, rosemary and garlic salt in a medium bowl. Add pecans and toss to coat. Spread in an even layer on a large rimmed baking sheet.

3. Bake, stirring every 15 minutes, until dry, about 45 minutes. Let cool completely before storing, about 30 minutes.

Tips

To make ahead: Store in an airtight container for up to 2 weeks.

5
APPENDICITIS DIET FOR CHILDREN

After undergoing appendix surgery, it's important for children to follow a specific dietary plan to aid recovery and prevent complications. A balanced diet rich in easily digestible foods like fruits, vegetables, lean proteins, and whole grains is recommended. Additionally, plenty of fluids, such as water and clear soups, help maintain hydration. Avoiding heavy or spicy foods, as well as foods that may cause gas or bloating, can support a smoother recovery process for the children.

Recovering from appendix surgery requires special attention to your child's diet to promote healing and restore energy levels. Here's a detailed guide on what foods to include, avoid, and other helpful tips during your child's recovery, in consultation with a pediatric surgeon.

Clear Liquids:

Encourage your child to start with clear liquids like water, broth, apple juice, and clear, non-carbonated beverages after surgery.

These help prevent dehydration and are gentle on the digestive system.

Easy-to-Digest Foods:

As your child progresses, introduce easy-to-digest foods like plain crackers, toast, rice, and applesauce.

These foods are gentle on the stomach and help in the healing process.

Protein-Rich Foods:

Incorporate protein-rich foods like lean meats, poultry, fish, eggs, and dairy products into your child's diet.

Protein is essential for tissue repair and overall recovery.

Fiber-Rich Foods:

Gradually introduce high-fiber foods like fruits, vegetables, whole grains, and legumes to promote healthy digestion.

Fiber helps prevent constipation, a common issue after surgery.

Hydration:

Ensure your child stays hydrated by drinking plenty of water throughout the day.

Proper hydration supports the healing process and overall well-being.

Avoid Irritating Foods:

Stay away from spicy, greasy, and processed foods that may irritate the digestive system.

Opt for bland, easily digestible options to prevent discomfort.

Small, frequent meals:

Encourage your child to have small, frequent meals throughout the day rather than large, heavy meals.

This aids in digestion and prevents overloading the system.

Consult with a healthcare provider:

Always consult with your child's healthcare provider or pediatric doctor for personalized dietary recommendations post-appendix surgery. They can provide appropriate advice based on your child's specific needs and recovery progress. By following these dietary guidelines, you can help support your child's recovery after appendix surgery and promote their overall well-being. Remember, patience and a balanced diet are key elements in aiding your child's journey to a speedy recovery.

Conclusion:

Ensuring proper nutrition plays an important role in aiding children's recovery after appendix surgery. A diet rich in clear liquids, easy-to-digest foods, protein, and Fiber helps promote healing and prevent complications such as dehydration and constipation. It's important to avoid irritating foods and opt for small, frequent meals to support digestion. Consulting with healthcare providers for personalized dietary guidance is paramount. By adhering to these dietary recommendations, parents can assist their children in achieving a smooth and speedy recovery, fostering their overall well-being during this crucial period.

Transitioning to the Appendicitis Diet

Expect a few weeks of recovery from an appendectomy — or longer if your appendix burst. To help your body heal:

- **Limit your activity.** If your appendectomy was done laparoscopically, limit your activity for 3 to 5 days. If you had an open appendectomy, limit your activity for 10 to 14 days. Always ask your healthcare team about limits on your activity and when you can resume your typical activities after surgery.

- **Support your abdomen when you cough.** To help reduce pain, place a pillow over your belly and apply pressure before you cough, laugh or move.

- **Contact your healthcare team if your pain medicines aren't helping.** Being in pain puts extra stress on your body and slows the healing process. If you're still in pain despite taking your pain medicines, call a member of your healthcare team.

- **Get up and move when you're ready.** Start slowly and increase your activity as you feel able. Begin with short walks.

- **Sleep when tired.** As your body heals, you may find that you feel more tired than usual. Take it easy and rest when you need to.

- **Discuss returning to work or school with your healthcare team.** You can return to work when you feel ready. Children may be able to return to school less than a week after surgery. They should wait 2 to 4 weeks to return to certain activities, such as gym classes or sports.

Alternative medicine

You will be prescribed medicines to help you control pain after your appendectomy. Other treatments, when used with your medicines, can help control pain. Ask your healthcare team about safe options, such as:

- Distracting activities, such as listening to music and talking with friends, that take your mind off your pain. Distraction can be especially effective with children.

- Practicing meditation to help calm the body. Also be sure to get plenty of rest.

Preparing for your appointment

Make an appointment with a member of your healthcare team if you have abdominal pain. If you have appendicitis, you'll likely be hospitalized and referred to a surgeon to remove your appendix.

What you can do

When you make the appointment, ask if there's anything you need to do in advance, such as fasting before having a specific test. Make a list of:

- **Your symptoms,** including any that might not seem related to the reason for your appointment.

- **Key personal information,** including major stresses, recent life changes and family medical history.

- **All medicines, vitamins or other supplements** you take and the doses.

- **Questions to ask** your healthcare team.

Take a family member or friend along, if possible, to help you remember the information you're given.

For appendicitis, some basic questions to ask include:

- Do I have appendicitis?
- Will I need more tests?
- What else could I have besides appendicitis?
- Do I need surgery and, if so, how soon?
- What are the risks of appendix removal?
- How long will I need to stay in the hospital after surgery?
- How long will recovery take?

- How soon after surgery can I go back to work?

- Can you tell whether my appendix has burst?

Don't hesitate to ask other questions.

What to expect from your doctor

You are likely to be asked several questions, such as:

- When did your abdominal pain begin?

- Where does it hurt?

- Has the pain moved?

- How bad is your pain?

- What makes your pain more severe?

- What helps relieve your pain?

- Do you have a fever?

- Do you feel nauseated?

- What other symptoms do you have?

www.ingramcontent.com/pod-product-compliance
Lightning Source LLC
Chambersburg PA
CBHW052248220526
45471CB00001B/238